COVID-19
& ITS CHALLENGES
Is India Future Ready?

COVID-19

& ITS CHALLENGES

Is India Future Ready?

Edited by

VK Ahluwalia & Amrita Jash

Centre for Land Warfare Studies

PENTAGON PRESS LLP

The Centre for Land Warfare Studies (CLAWS), New Delhi, is an autonomous Think Tank dealing with contemporary issues of national security and conceptual aspects of land warfare, including conventional and sub-conventional conflicts and terrorism. CLAWS conducts research that is futuristic in outlook and policy-oriented in approach.

CLAWS Vision: To establish CLAWS as a leading Think Tank in policy formulation on Land Warfare, National Security and Strategic Issues.

Centre for Land Warfare Studies
RPSO Complex, Parade Road, Delhi Cantt, New Delhi-110010
Phone: 011-25691308 • CLAWS ARMY NO : 33098 • Fax: 011-25692347
email: landwarfare@gmail.com • website: www.claws.in

First Published in 2020

ISBN 978-93-90095-02-5

Published by
PENTAGON PRESS LLP
206, Peacock Lane, Shahpur Jat,
New Delhi-110049
Phones: 011-64706243, 26491568
Telefax: 011-26490600
email: rajan@pentagonpress.in
website: www.pentagon-press.com

Printed at Aegean Offset Printers, Greater Noida, U.P.

To Those Who Inspired to Shape a
Better Future For India

CONTENTS

General NC Vij
PVSM, UYSM, AVSM (Retd)
Hony Col of the DOGRA Regt & DOGRA Scouts

Former -
*Chief of the Army Staff
*Founder Vice Chairman
National Disaster Management Authority
*Director
Vivekanand International Foundation

House No - 4500A, Sector-23A
Gurgaon (Haryana)
PIN - 122017
Ph: 0124-4364500
E-mail: gncvij@gmail.com

FOREWORD

The COVID-19 pandemic has become one of the biggest global tragedies of all times. It has changed the old narratives of national security which delved mainly on the 'borders'. The emerging new security paradigm is gravely challenged by 'non-traditional security' issues, such as infectious diseases that are not limited by borders. The raging impact of the pandemic on 'life and livelihood' has manifested in the form of demographic losses, health care collapse and economic downturn. These aspects have made it imminent to look beyond the traditional understanding of a 'nation's security'. It has become very clear that a nation can survive only if 'human security' is taken well care of.

After five months since it outbreak from January 2020, COVID-19 has made major powers such as United States, China, EU and others to realise that arms race alone cannot tackle all contingencies. The bigger quandary is: How to fight an invisible enemy? This has caused a reality check, pushing for the old security matrix to undergo a transformation. Although no country has been spared from the scourge of the virus, India, unlike the other major powers, has succeeded in keeping the rate of infection as well as the mortality rate comparatively low despite its highly dense population of 1.3 billions.

With the largest nationwide lockdown, India does merit attention for its handling of the pandemic. However, this does not make India an exception from the grave challenges attached to the COVID-19. With the economy hit hard, the lockdown has highlighted the misery of India's large migrant workforce, lack of health care facilities, connectivity issues highlighting the shortcomings in the plans of the Centre and the States for timely action. However, not all is Grey.

The pandemic has also provided India with an opportunity to elevate its status, display its 'responsible image' through its global outreach efforts to other countries with medical aid, food supplies, export of medicines such as hydroxychloroquine and paracetamol as well as safely evacuating, the Indians from abroad. Towards this goal, India's Armed Forces have displayed a hands on approach despite the challenges of travel bans. What has caught the eye of the world, is India's global approach in fighting the pandemic as well as leading by setting a personal example.

The need of the hour calls for a "Re-Think and Refining" India's national security issues and policies in practice- both at home and abroad, it is time to push the security envelope, rather than fold it further.

Towards this aim, this book makes it a veritable read both in terms of understanding and assessment of what lies ahead for India, as commonly called in the 'post-COVID world'. Offering an Indian perspective to the unfolding pandemic situation, the volume deals with addressing the impact on India's national security from social, political, economic, military, environment, and strategic perspectives. With its all-encompassing outlook, this book by CLAWS makes a timely and valuable contribution towards providing a blueprint to 'What can be done' by laying out an astute list of recommendations.

CLAWS with its proactive approach in pitching this topical piece has indeed set an example of fulfilling the aim of Think Tanks of 'providing a nation with a timely guidance'. Furthermore, the study aids the key objective set out by India's National Security Advisor, Mr Ajit Doval in studying the impact of COVID-19 on India's national security. Being the first of its kind, this book by CLAWS compliments the phrase - 'A Stitch in Time Saves Nine'!

This book will be valuable for all policy makers, economic and strategic analysts, academia, medical fraternity, essential services' personnel and civil and security personnel alike.

I will like to convey my deepest compliments to the CLAWS for this novel output.

New Delhi
12 June 2020

NC Vij
General

ACKNOWLEDGEMENTS

A book of this kind is the culmination of many people's goodwill, conscientious efforts and above all, a dedicated commitment towards nation building. The main objective behind the pursuit has been the 'uncertain times' and the 'need to do' something about it. When India and its people are fighting a deadly virus, this book grew out of the necessity. This was an unforeseen consequence which will be beneficial for years to come. The most important part of this journey were its challenges, but the strength to fight the odds came from the people who showed faith against all odds.

Such an arduous task in the uncertain times of the lockdown has been possible solely due to the collaborative and sincere commitment of those who helped to bring this book to fruition. At the foremost, a note of high appreciation goes to each of the authors—Ms Kanchana Ramanujam, Dr. Manjari Singh, Col RS Sandhu, Brig Akhelesh Bhargava, Air Commodore Ashminder Singh Bahal, Maj Gen PK Chakravorty and Lt Gen Rakesh Sharma, in making a valuable contribution that shaped the book in a timely manner. In particular, we would extend a note of gratitude to our Deputy Directors, Col HS Burn and Col Amit Hajela, for their support and coordinated efforts to pursue this project despite the odd times. A special gratitude note to Ms Shreya Das Barman for her sincere efforts from the very beginning, from getting the beautiful cover for the book to that of making things fall into place in the most timely way. Her hard work and sincerity are highly appreciated.

A special note of thanks to General NC Vij, former Chief of the Army Staff, whose encouragement helped in the endeavour and his Foreword has laid the foundation for the book. A note of high appreciation is extended to Ambassador PS Raghavan, Chairman, National Security Advisory Board, Ambassador Vijay Gokhale, former Foreign Secretary, and Lt Gen Devraj Anbu, former Vice Chief of the Army Staff, for their valuable thoughts about the book.

A sincere thanks to Ms Tejusvi Shukla, Ms Anashwara Ashok, Mr Raghunandan, Mrs Priyadarshini Shetty, Lt Col Poshuk Ahluwalia, Col Himanshu Kataria, Col Sunil Gupta, and Col Ranjan Prabhu for their valuable insights.

No study of this nature could have materialised without the significant institutional support, a special note of thanks to Mr Dharmender Bansiwal, Nitesh Khandelwal and the administrative staff of CLAWS for their tacit support. Lastly, a special note of gratitude to each one and all at CLAWS for their belief, support, and encouragement to pursue this timely book.

Although the subject is dynamic, it has been our earnest endeavour to publish an editorial and scholarly book, based on the events that unfolded until the month of June 2020; as also to crystal gaze beyond the horizon and to shape a secure and brighter India.

VK Ahluwalia & Amrita Jash

ABBREVIATIONS

ADB	Asian Development Bank
AFMS	Armed Forces Medical Service
AI	Artificial Intelligence
AIDS	Acquired Immune Deficiency Syndrome
API	Active Pharmaceutical Ingredient
BRI	Belt and Road Initiative
BTWC	Biological and Toxin Weapons Convention
BS-IV	Bharat Stage Four
BS-VI	Bharat Stage Six
CCTV	Closed Circuit Television
CII	Confederation of Indian Industry
CIL	Coal India Limited
CMIE	Centre for Monitoring Indian Economy
CNP	Comprehensive National Power
COAS	Chief of the Army Staff
COMCASA	Communications Compatibility and Security Agreement
COVID-19	Coronavirus Disease 2019
CPC	Communist Party of China
CPEC	China-Pakistan Economic Corridor
DIB	Defence Industrial Base
DMA	Department of Military Affairs
DRDO	Defence Research and Development Organisation
ECS	East China Sea
EU	European Union
FATF	Financial Action Task Force

FCI	Food Corporation of India
FDI	Foreign Direct Investment
FICCI	Federation of Indian Chambers of Commerce and Industry
FMCG	Fast Moving Consumer Goods
FSSAI	Food Safety and Standards Authority of India
FWO	Frontier Works Organization
FY	Financial Year
G11	Group of 11
G20	Group of 20
GDP	Gross Development Product
GHGs	Green House Gases
GHI	Global Hunger Index
GPS	Global Positioning System
GSQR	General Staff Qualitative Requirement
HCQ	Hydroxychloroquine
HDCU	High Dependency Care Units
HDFC	Housing Development Finance Corporation
HDR	Human Development Report
HUL	Hindustan Unilever Limited
IACCS	Integrated Air Command and Control System
IB	International Border
ICC	Indian Chamber of Commerce
ICMR	Indian Council of Medical Research
ICU	Intensive Care Unit
IDSA	Institute of Defence Studies and Analyses
IFF	Identification Friend or Foe
IIT	Indian Institute of Technology
IIM	Indian Institute of Management
ILO	Intrenational Labour Organization
IMA	Indian Medical Association
IMF	International Monetary Fund
INMAS	Institute of Nuclear Medicine and Allied Sciences
IOR	Indian Ocean Region
IPCC	Intergovernmental Panel on Climate Change

IPM	Indian Pharmaceutical Market
IRNSS	Indian Regional Navigation Satellite System
ISRO	Indian Space Research Organisation
IT	Information Technology
IW	Information Warfare
J&K	Jammu and Kashmir
LEMOA	Logistics Exchange Memorandum of Agreement
LoC	Line of Control
LAC	Line of Actual Control
M&M	Mahindra and Mahindra
MCI	Ministry of Commerce and Industry
MDG	Millennium Development Goal
MEA	Ministry of External Affairs
MERS-CoV	Middle East Respiratory Syndrome Coronavirus
MHA	Ministry of Home Affairs
MMT	MakeMy Trip
MoD	Ministry of Defence
MRO	Maintenance, Repair and Overhaul
MSME	Micro, Small and Medium Enterprises
MSP	Minimum Support Price
NCDC	National Centre for Disease Control
NDMA	National Disaster Management Authority
NDRF	National Disaster Relief Force
NPC	National People's Congress
NSCS	National Security Council Secretariat
NSE	National Stock Exchange
NSG	Nuclear Suppliers Group
NSN	National Security Number
NSS	National Security Strategy
NTRO	National Technical Research Organisation
NTS	Non-Traditional Security
OECD	Organisation for Economic Co-operation and Development
OFB	Ordnance Factory Board
PDS	Public Distribution System

PKR	Pakistani Rupees
PLA	People's Liberation Army
PMO	Prime Minister's Office
PN3	Press Note 3
PPP	Purchasing Power Parity
QR	Quick Response
R&D	Research and Development
RBI	Reserve Bank of India
RFID	Radio Frequency Identification
RIL	Reliance Industries Limited
SAARC	South Asian Association for Regional Cooperation
SARS	Severe Acute Respiratory Syndrome
SARS-CoV-2	Severe Acute Respiratory Syndrome Coronavirus 2
SCS	South China Sea
SDG	Sustainable Development Goal
SEZ	Special Economic Zone
SIPRI	Stockholm International Peace Research Institute
SMET	Science, Technology, Engineering and Mathematics
SOP	Standard Operating Procedure
UK	United Kingdom
UN	United Nations
UNCTAD	United Nations Conference on Trade and Development
UNDESA	United Nations Department for Economic and Social Affairs
UNDP	United Nations Development Programme
UNSC	United Nations Security Council
USA	United States of America
UT	Union Territory
WHA	World Health Assembly
WHO	World Health Organization

ILLUSTRATIONS

Figures

Table

INTRODUCTION

"The COVID-19 crisis gave us lessons [...]. It is from this lesson - Atmanirbhar Bharat (self-reliant India) campaign has started. It is time for bold decisions and bold investments, and not for conservative approaches. This also is the time to move from command and control economy to plug-and-play and to build a competitive global supply chain".

— Prime Minister Narendra Modi,
ICC Plenary Session, 11 June 2020.

The essence of the above statement by Prime Minister Modi highlights the need to turn the COVID-19 pandemic into an 'opportunity' for India- calling for an '*Atmanirbhar Bharat*'. This very aspect contextualises the central theme of the book that aims to address the key query: *Is India Future Ready?*

With the world put to disorder by the invisible virus named 'Severe Acute Respiratory Syndrome Coronavirus 2' (SARS-CoV-2), India's such an optimistic outlook is driven by the realisation of the 'new normal'- as the old ways of thinking cannot help draw a balance between 'life and livelihood'. India reported its first case on 30 January and the first nationwide lockdown was imposed on 24 March. Since then COVID-19 has exposed the perils of inequality, the social and economic disparity, and the widening cracks resulting from the attempt to maintain stability- both internal and external. In this perspective, the rapidly changing dynamics require India to realign its national priorities and interests – calling for a total 'transformation'. Wherein, the need of the hour lies in re-defining India's national policy at all levels- social, economic, political and military. Having emerged as the biggest global tragedy of the 21st century, COVID-19 has significantly challenged the old narrative that defined security, as the new concerns are not limited by borders.

As the virus continues to spread and drawing from the past experiences of Severe Acute Respiratory Syndrome (SARS) and Middle East Respiratory Syndrome (MERS-CoV), the concerns over the emergence of a second wave of COVID-19 has been further accentuated. With no clear end in sight and the raging scale and intensity of infection, the fact remains that the virus may prevail for long. In view of this, with sovereignty still at the apex of national interest, the pandemic with its devastative impact in terms of demographic loss, health care collapse and economic downturn has raised skepticism over the 'state-centric' approach to security. Against the collateral damage caused by COVID-19, old security calculations call for a re-boot. Thus, making it imperative to re-look at India's 'vision to be' in the post pandemic order.

In this perspective, the book aims to address three key questions: First, How has the definition of 'national security' been impacted by the challenges posed by the pandemic? Second, What factors need to dominate India's new national security and interest calculus? And finally, What will define India's post pandemic outlook? In examining these key queries, the central objective of this timely volume lies in deriving recommendations for 'making India future ready' in the post-COVID world.

As befits a study of such a comprehensive nature, this book makes multiple arguments and sub arguments; however, the overarching thesis is centred on offering an Indian perspective to 'COVID-19 and its challenges'. Given the vastness of the subject of enquiry, the scope of the book is limited and is mainly concentrated on analysing some of the core issues of concern. In doing so, the book is structured into nine chapters- each pertaining to a key theme. With its holistic approach, the volume makes a comprehensive study embedded in assessing the core aspects pertaining to: the need to revisit the security debate by prioritising 'human security' and environmental security' in the national security calculus; aiming for sustainability in drawing the right balance between 'means, ways and ends' in national policy; making India self-reliant at all sectors; taking a proactive and leading role in global decision-making; the need for re-appraisal of India's military thinking and strategy; the evolving role of the Indian Armed Forces with special emphasis on biological warfare and; finally, technology as the new state-of-the-art for India to master, in stepping up the internal and external security bracket.

In combatting a pandemic effectively, some of the key words are: good leadership, solidarity, trust and cooperation at all levels, compassion and an innovative approach to find implementable solutions. To overcome the challenges in a democratic federal structure with a huge population base, support and trust of the people remain central in winning the battle against the pandemic. Owing to this multi-dimensional perspective, the final chapter of the book denominated as *Making India Future Ready* is where the solution lies, in the form of a blueprint for India's recovery process amidst the crisis. While the Indian Government aims at taking the right measures; however, the biggest challenge is that of acting with a 'sense of emergency' and ensuring 'proper timely implementation' of the policies. Therefore, the need of the hour lies in bridging these existing gaps.

The time is of essence and India cannot wait any longer for its ship to arrive. Hence, the calling is: ***Think Wisely, Act Responsibly and March Ahead Tall!***

1

India's National Security: Old Threats Imbalanced with New Challenges

VK Ahluwalia

COVID-19 has brought the world to its undeclared 'Third World War', caused not by any kinetic action, but by an invisible enemy. Calling for a global health emergency, the coronavirus outbreak has emerged as a deadly weapon of mass destruction, bringing the world to a standstill. The world is faced with a grave challenge of bringing the pandemic under control and drawing a balance between 'life and livelihood'.

The pandemic has impacted the developed countries (USA, UK, Italy, France, Spain, and others) the most, highlighting their inability to effectively deal with its severity. The developing and underdeveloped countries are also facing the consequences due to their fragility resulting from weak economies, high population density, lower literacy levels, inadequate medical facilities, and insufficient infrastructure; thus, the virus is not selective in its impact. What calls for this global plight?

In the past, the lessons from the experiences of two respiratory epidemics—the 2002-03 SARS[1] that started in China, and the 2012-13 MERS-CoV[2] that was identified in Saudi Arabia, were both loud and clear. Some of the lessons drawn from SARS suggested the following recommendations: the need for an early and transparent reporting by individuals and countries to minimise both infections and mortality;

sharing known information and protective measures; global surveillance mechanism, reporting and the key role of the World Health Organization (WHO); coordinating scientific investigations; psychological support of health care workers; system of financial incentives and international censures; all laboratories with the pathogen should review their protocols for strict adherence to procedures; programmes for counselling its healthcare workers who are at risk of infection and death; the role of information technology to communicate; and imposing quarantine with care and compassion.[3]

In view of the failure in handling the COVID-19 pandemic, a key query that demands significant attention is: Did we really learn some lessons from SARS and MERS-CoV, and did we implement them to avert future crisis? The answer is 'No', as the world was deeply unprepared in combating the catastrophe of COVID-19. For the reality lies in the fact that so far countries were mainly focused on the military aspect of security. This is evident from the increasing global military expenditure, which reached US$ 1,917 billion in 2019—the largest annual increase in a decade.[4]

In this perspective, COVID-19 has brought to the fore the need to strike a correct balance between addressing the external and internal threats to the health care of populations from infectious diseases and environmental degradation. In addition, the crisis has made it essential for major powers and their governments to act responsive- both towards its people and the world at large. For if China had given an early warning, a transparent reporting of the Wuhan epidemic as well as given precautionary measures to be adopted—such a forewarning to the world would have helped bring the pandemic under reasonable control. A repercussion of which is witnessed in the global spread of the virus which, as per WHO, has infected 10,185,374 people in 213 countries, and has claimed 503,862 lives, as on 30 June 2020.[5] While in India alone, 566,840 people have been infected, and 16,893 have died due to the virus, as on 30 June 2020.[6] What is noteworthy is that globally, since end of May, there has been a sharp increase in the confirmed cases of COVID-19; however, in India, the spike in cases was witnessed only after 2 June and the 'recovery rate of the total confirmed' cases have also shown progressive improvement in India. The details of the virus spread across the world and in India are outlined in Figures 1.1 and 1.2.

Figure 1.1: Trend of COVID-19 outbreak in the World (until 30 June 2020)

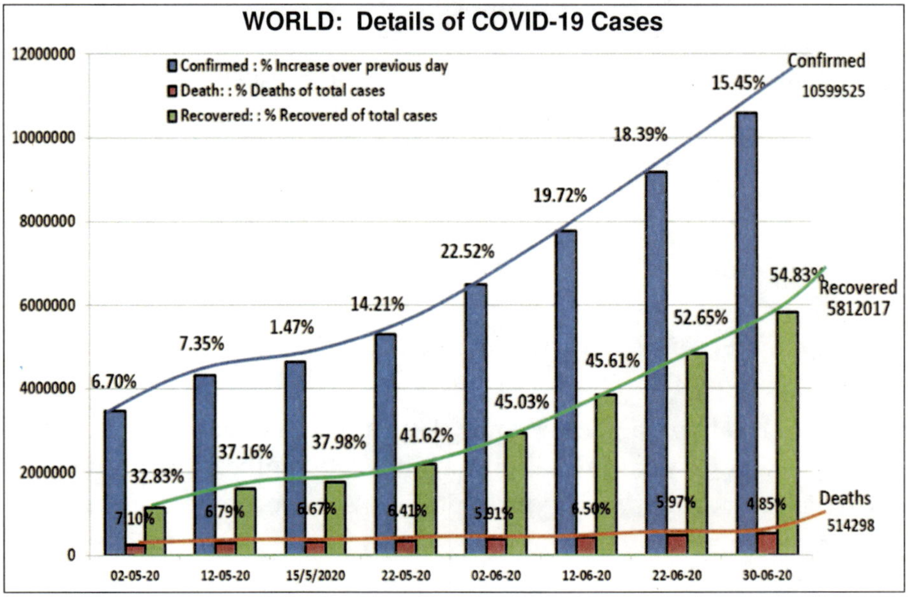

Source: Prepared by Author with data available at Worldometer.[7]

Figure 1.2: Trend of COVID-19 outbreak in India (until 30 June 2020)

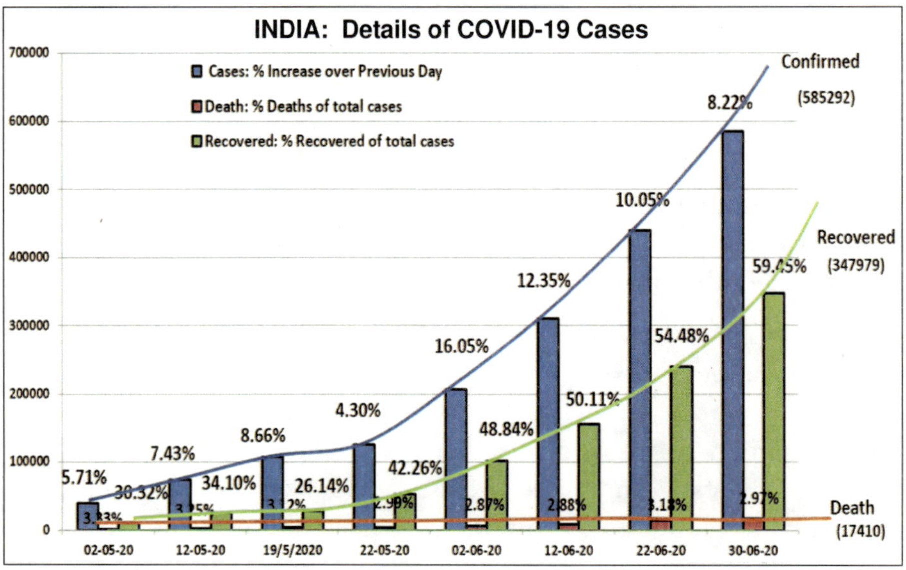

Source: Prepared by Author with data available at Worldometer.[8]

Keeping the global impact of COVID-19 as the backdrop, the present chapter seeks to examine the pandemic largely from a national security perspective. In doing so, the chapter will mainly focus on India's national security, which will be studied from a two-fold perspective: the politico-economic-strategic environment as impacted by COVID-19; and the criticality of non-traditional threats to India's national security. The crux of the chapter lies in assessing the threats, challenges and opportunities that are likely to shape India's national security strategy in the post-pandemic world order.

Changing Scope of National Security: *Not Just Traditional, But also Non-Traditional*

In the aftermath of the Cold War, with the phenomenon of globalisation at play, the world witnessed a spike in intrastate conflicts, predominantly in Africa and Asia. Mainly prompted by socio-economic disparities, sectarian, ethnic and religious divides, and fragile governance systems; these acts of violence brought to the surface the travesty of human suffering in terms of heavy casualties, loss of livelihood, human displacement, and mass migrations. This aspect of 'human security' was first highlighted in the United Nations Development Programme's (UNDP) landmark 1994 Human Development Report (HDR), entitled *New Dimensions of Human Security*[9] that introduced a new concept of human security, equating security with people rather than territories with sustainable development or arms. Calling human security *"people-centred,"* the Report categorically stated: "It is concerned with how people live and breathe in a society, how freely they exercise their many choices, how much access they have to market and social opportunities, and whether they live in conflict or in peace".[10]

This reflected a shift from the traditional concept of security that had mainly been narrowly interpreted in the fixed contours of security of territory from external aggression; as protection of national interests in foreign policy; or as global security resulting from a nuclear threat, more nation-state-centric than people-oriented. National security has been mainly defined in geo-political terms, limited to relationships among nation-states mainly dealing with issues of deterrence, balance of power and military strategy. This then guides the formulation of a country's national security strategy (NSS). However, with the rapid changes in the nature and intensity of the security environment, the dividing line between internal and external security threats is increasingly getting blurred.[11]

Defying the accustomed thinking of national security in terms of 'military threats', Richard H. Ullman called such a perception as "doubly misleading".[12] Ullman argues that it draws attention away from the non-military threats that promise to undermine the stability of many nations during the years ahead and also presupposes that threats arising from outside a state are somehow more dangerous to its security than threats that arise within it.[13] This argument stands justified, given COVID-19 is a perfect example of a 'non-military' threat or as commonly denoted a 'non-traditional security' (NTS) threat that has affected the entire world, posing a threat to the survival of states and its people.

What makes a 'non-traditional threat'? Mely Caballero-Anthony in the book entitled *An Introduction to Non-Traditional Security Studies: A Transnational Approach* defines it as challenges to the survival and well-being of peoples and states that arise primarily out of non-military sources, such as climate change, cross-border environmental degradation and resource depletion, infectious diseases, natural disasters, irregular migration, food shortages, people smuggling, drug trafficking, and other forms of transnational crime.[14]

In contrast to the traditional understanding, NTS comprises issues related to international terrorism, trans-national organised crime, environmental security, illegal migration, energy security and human security.[15] Such non-military threats are mainly characterised as being transnational in nature, defined in political and socio-economic terms, caused by societal and political instability and human-induced disturbances that essentially require regional and multilateral cooperation and that referent of security is no longer just the state.[16] According to HDR of 1994, the seven essential dimensions of human security are: economic security, food security, health security, environmental security, personal security, community security, and political security.[17] To note, in the past few decades, human security has been faced with the risks borne from mainly environmental degradation, widespread human displacements, internal armed conflicts and increased zoonotic transmissions due to human-animal interface.

According to a WHO report, between 2011-2017, 1,307 epidemics were recorded across 172 countries worldwide.[18] With 'infectious diseases' increasingly becoming a potent non-traditional threat as seen in the outbreak of SARS, MERS-CoV and now, COVID-19, the human security aspect merits significant attention in the larger ambit of national security. Threats to human security are no longer just personal or local or national, but are transnational and beyond regional boundaries. These are ever evolving with changes in the nature and severity of the threat that is explained as follows:

First, the priority of NTS differs from region to region and country to country; wherein, mostly economic and environmental security figure prominently in every country's agenda. For instance, in China, the region-wise priority of NTS issues include economic security, ecological security, information security, population security; three "evil forces" of religious extremism, separatism and terrorism; drug trafficking, AIDS, small-scale weapon transaction, pirate rampancy, oil tanker leakage, money trafficking, refugee and illegal immigrants.[19] This perspective is applicable to other states and regions as well. In addition, other dimensions like water security, energy security, cyber and information security and security from natural disasters also affect human security.

Second, most of the NTS, including COVID-19 are linked and are interdependent on each other in some form or the other. Economic, environmental, and social security plays a vital role in providing a secure and good quality of life to people. If developing and under-developed countries have a sustained economic growth, they can at least look after the survival requirements of their people in terms of food, water, health, job opportunities and others.

Third, given the increased hyperactive urbanisation, population growth, industrialisation, several thermal power plants and high energy consumption, it is evident that urban areas are major contributors to the emission of greenhouse gases (GHGs), issues of climate change, global warming, water degradation, air pollution, environmental pollution, and waste disposal. These are detrimental to the health of human beings and animals, and gravely affect the survival of the natural ecosystem.

Fourth, outbreak of epidemics/pandemics affects both social-economic-political security situations within a country and interstate relations. Depending upon the severity of NTS threats such as COVID-19, it can also be identified as a catalyst that can trigger tension and a conflict situation within states and region.

Time to Reset India's National Security Priorities: *Health as the Survival Need*

As compared to traditional threats, the NTS threats are posing greater challenges to human security and the well-being of the people. With COVID-19, this thesis has been significantly validated. What makes health security integral to national security?

First, health security is one of the most important survival needs of the people as testified by the severity and impact of COVID-19. It has also brought to the fore other life-threatening challenges posed by environmental degradation. As noted by Douglas Broom, air pollution has emerged as the biggest health hazard among the developing countries. For instance, it is noted that six of the world's 10 most polluted cities are in India that kill 1.25 million people in India every year and that New Delhi has the worst air pollution of any capital city.[20] A report by the UN suggests that 45 per cent of India's children are stunted and that 600,000 children under five die each year, largely because of inadequate water supply and poor sanitation.[21]

What is noteworthy is that despite its growing vulnerabilities caused by air and water, India has not given due importance and seriousness to address these issues in its annual budget, which has increased from Rs. 2,658 crore to Rs. 3,100 crore in FY 20-21.[22] However, this sum is too little to address the increasing environmental security concerns which affects human health and the natural eco-system. In view of this, it can be argued that if survival needs of the people (water, food and health care) are affected by environmental degradation, atmospheric pollution or biological factors resulting into infectious diseases like SARS, MERS-CoV and COVID-19; this could trigger social unrest, as already noted in the distress caused to over 120 million migrant labour population[23] under the lockdown.

Second, besides biological hazards, other threats such as environmental security, energy security, cyber security, displacement, and mass migration of people also have the potential to develop into traditional security threats and challenges in the future. Therefore, the state and the international community must address all threats that travel across regions, beyond political boundaries like virus, bacteria, bioagents; atmospheric and environmental pollution; and climate change that impact humans and all living organs. This makes it imperative for India to address environmental issues with sincerity and must promote a long-term perspective plan for renewable energy to minimise environmental degradation. This requires the need to boost and improve the healthcare facilities across India and make significant investments in R&D to prevent the health care from getting overwhelmed under a crisis, as noted under COVID-19, or the cases affected by air and water pollution every year.

To support healthcare against pandemics, India needs to depart from old standalone practices of quarantine and social distancing and instead, optimise technology-enabled systems. This will help aid a 'non-contact' prevention and control measure by using facial recognition and contact tracing through smart phone technology and thermal imaging cameras in public places, based on artificial intelligence (AI) and big data available. The use of technology-enabled systems in handling the pandemic was successful in a few countries, such as Taiwan, China, South Korea, and others. This is primarily because their whole management strategy revolved around availability of a database of their population and an effective system of communicating policies, guidelines, and monitoring each case. It facilitated surveillance, testing, social distancing, tracing contact history, timely treatment, and others.

In case of India, some of the biggest problems that have spiked the cases are: lack of data of the population; ineffective assessment methodology to monitor cases; inadequate medical facilities, staff and infrastructure; high density of population; and high percentage of people living in slums and ghettos.[24] In addition, India's total expenditure on healthcare is miniscule as compared to the size of the population. For instance, the Centre's and states' health budgets for FY20 was Rs. 2.6 trillion, accounting for 1.29 per cent of the GDP, as opposed to 1.02 per cent of the GDP in 2016-17.[25] This includes establishment expenditure comprising salaries and gross budgetary support to various medical schemes, institutions, and hospitals. India's total healthcare spending (out-of-pocket and public), comprising 3.6 per cent of the GDP, as suggested by OECD, is way lower than that of other countries.[26] Besides, India spends the least among BRICS countries. Therefore, India needs to raise its health expenditure as a percentage of its GDP. On balance, India needs to do enormous work to be 'Future Ready'.

India's Security Roulette: *Balancing Concerns with Strategy*

India, by virtue of its geographical location, demographic dividend, and fair reserves of natural resources, has a significant geo-strategic advantage. Situated at the crossroads of regions like West Asia, Central Asia, Southeast Asia, with attendant advantages and its peninsula projects into the Indian Ocean Region (IOR), provides it with a boon to command a vast expanse of the Indian Ocean and the critical sea lanes of communications.

With IOR acting as the maritime hub of the Indo-Pacific region, India enjoys the advantage of being a nodal centre of trade and communications, both in the continental and maritime domains. India can leverage its strategic advantage to increase its sphere of interest and influence in the new security architecture under the Indo-Pacific. However, to achieve its rightful place, India must first identify the prominent threats and challenges that it faces or is likely to face. India faces serious external threats, the prominent ones being from Pakistan, China, the Sino-Pakistan nexus, presence of nuclear armed states, maritime security and more recently, Nepal's claim to portions of Indian territory in Lipulekh area.

What looms large in India's security matrix is Pakistan, which itself is faced with several complex issues in the domains of politico-socio-economic, civil society, judiciary, and media. However, despite its own fragility, Pakistan continues to hinder India's national security interests. In doing so, Islamabad continues to play its religion card under 'Islam', promotes and maintains an anti-India stance both at the national and international levels, remains obsessed with Jammu and Kashmir (J&K) and its annexation by infusing a proxy war-cum-state sponsored terrorism in J&K, and initiates 'lone wolf terrorism' in other parts of India, all with an aim to destabilise New Delhi. In addition, even if Pakistan reduces its budgetary support to jihadis and terrorist groups due to the recession, but with support from China, it has been upgrading its military systems, information warfare systems, missiles, and nuclear arsenal capabilities. This, along with presence of Chinese security personnel in Gilgit-Baltistan region and along the China-Pakistan Economic Corridor (CPEC), makes the aspect of collusion a grave concern for India.

What significantly adds to India's security dilemma is the China factor, wherein the threat is increasingly getting magnified. China's rapid military modernisation, mechanisation, creation of theatre commands, streamlining of its command and control structures, improvement in its information and nuclear capabilities, has created an asymmetry with India in terms of capabilities. Its military capabilities refined with information and cyber capabilities are consistent with its military strategy and national security objectives. China aspires to become not only the world's largest nation in cyberspace but also among the most powerful. However, India's asymmetry with China is not just limited to the military capability but pervades in all domains: economy, science and technology, innovations, information and cyber capabilities, outer space, and nuclear capabilities. Notwithstanding, India has been one of the fastest growing large economies of the world. It has the potential to develop its economy to US$ five trillion in the next 4-5 years, as also upscale its comprehensive national power (CNP) to become a global power in the years ahead.

But increasingly China too is facing issues as witnessed in the slowdown of Beijing's economic growth over the last few years. Here, the big question is: Does economic slowdown affect China's great power ambitions? As Michael Beckley notes with caution: "When rising powers have suffered such slowdowns in the past, they become more repressive at home and more aggressive abroad" – as validated by examples from history.[27] Applying Beckley's assessment to the changed security scenario under COVID-19 and the resultant global recession, China could then be more aggressive in asserting its claims in areas of disputed territories as a tactic to divert the attention of the Chinese people. This would then remain an area of concern for the international community at large, and India in particular, as it shares an unresolved border with China. In the recent past, China has been aggressive on its periphery in the South China Sea (SCS), East China Sea (ECS), and the Taiwan Strait.

For India, the tension has already manifested with new military flare-ups being witnessed along the Line of Actual Control (LAC) in Eastern Ladakh and Sikkim. In early May, China's forces moved opposite Eastern Ladakh with multiple objectives, of which one of them was to re-align the LAC to serve its strategic interests. Faced with adversaries at two ends and hit by the pandemic, India's national security mainly has been focussed on the prevention and control of COVID-19. In doing so, India has been engaged in development of its healthcare and infrastructure reviving social, economic, and industrial sectors. But despite the pandemic, India cannot ignore its sovereignty and integrity issues; and thus, must remain operationally prepared for various contingencies against both China and Pakistan.

COVID-19 Creates the Tailspin: *What to Expect at Home and Abroad?*

It remains uncontested that globalisation has been one of most significant reasons why the coronavirus had spread to countries far beyond China at an alarming pace. Health emergency has been added with apprehensions, fear and psychological trauma, rapid changes in geo-political arena and economic disruptions, resulting in a social, economic, business, and political turmoil. Most notably, the pandemic has resulted in an economic emergency in turn resulting in recession-like conditions that have affected global trade, remittances, travel, tourism, hospitality industry, manufacturing industries, job opportunities, education, and global supply chains.

According to the International Monetary Fund (IMF) forecast of April 2020, the world economy was likely to suffer the worst financial crisis in 2020 since the Great Depression, and was likely to contract by 3 per cent (US$ 2.64 trillion) in 2020-21. As per IMF's *World Economic Outlook*, global growth is projected at minus 4.9 percent in 2020 -

1.9 percentage points below the April 2020 forecast.[28] Furthermore, it has projected a deeper 4.5 per cent contraction for India in 2020 than earlier estimated, citing a longer lockdown period and slower than anticipated recovery.[29] The COVID-19 pandemic has had a more negative impact on activity in the first half of 2020 than anticipated, and the recovery is projected to be more gradual than, as previously forecasted.[30] While the recovery in the labour markets will take some to stabilise.

Most countries, including India have announced stimulus packages to revive and sustain their economies. The impact of COVID-19 and the likewise growth projections are highlighted in Figure 1.3.

Figure 1.3: Impact of COVID-19: World Economy and Growth Projections for 2020

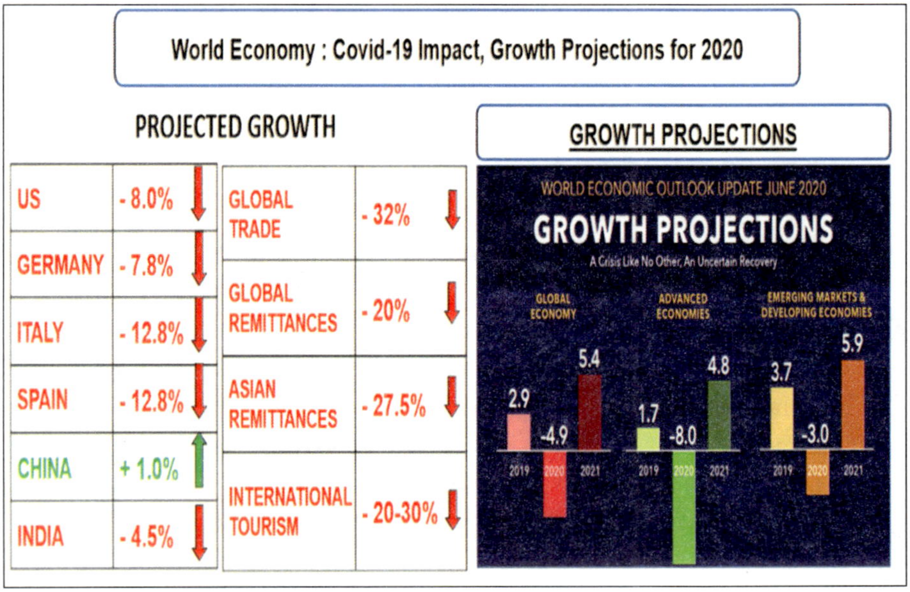

Source: Adapted from World Economic Outlook.[31]

Because of COVID-19, India's unemployment rate has increased 14.8 percentage points, rising to a high of 24 per cent in May 2020, as noted in Figure 1.4. The heightened number is difficult to overlook given it is one of the key indicators that determines prosperity in society and the security of a nation. This societal situation caused by economic fallout must be addressed on priority.

Figure 1.4: Monthly Unemployment Rate in India

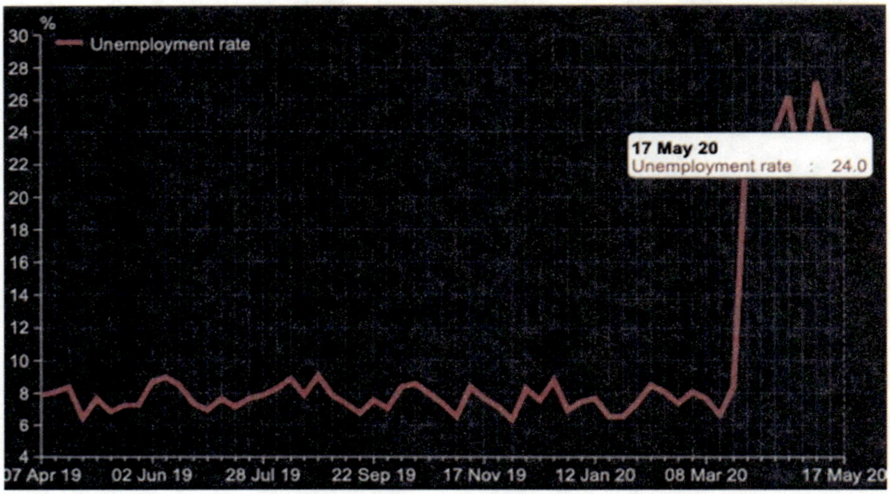

Source: Adapted from Centre for Monitoring Indian Economy Pvt Ltd (CMIE) Survey.[32]

Envisaged Trends and Changes

Given the prevailing geo-situation and the tension prevailing between the US and China, the world is likely to witness re-alignment in the geo-political, economic, and strategic domains in the near future. It becomes imperative to understand the changes that can be expected in the post-COVID world. While the priorities are likely to revolve around revival of economic growth, health care and building infrastructure, environmental protection and sustainable development, the changes are likely to be witnessed in areas such as: First, stalled globalisation will manifest increased protectionism, opting for self-reliance and self-sufficiency, enhanced emphasis on regionalism and sub-regionalism, and focus on domestic production and market consumption. Second, severe disruptions in global value and supply chain systems will lead to diversification and building of regional and sub-regional based supply chain systems. Third, prevention of disasters with 'trans-boundary and trans-regions spread features' like epidemics, infectious diseases, and natural disasters caused by environmental degradation will require a coordinated response mechanism, both at the global and regional levels. Fourth, in addition to other priorities, developing countries would also focus on the survival needs of people, addressing problems of migrant labour, displaced people, and poverty reduction. Fifth, new norms of working culture will come into force, such as work from home (WFH), and virtual interactions/conferences/seminars. Sixth, due to recession and resultant high unemployment rates, there could be an increase in social unrest, armed conflicts, terrorism, and organised crime. Seventh, a few hegemonic countries can exploit the crisis situation by laying claims to territories which do not legally belong to them. A case in point is China's aggressiveness against its neighbours on its periphery, at both sea and on land. Eighth, during the pandemic and the resultant severe economic downturn/recession, the term 'Frugal Innovations,' an old concept, would be revived with vigour. It aims to provide affordable consumer goods and services to the people at large, by adopting innovative measures.

However, the pandemic with its spread, human suffering, and impact on the economy would have a lasting impact on the emerging new world order. A shift would be witnessed in the balance of power, geo-politico-economic-strategic environment, globalisation, trade and supply chains, healthcare, mental and psychological wellbeing of people amongst others. As for the last three decades, the USA continued to remain the sole superpower in the world with China, emerging as the next close competitor of the USA. However, the circumstances of the pandemic have jolted the heavyweights of both the USA and China. The post-pandemic world will witness a re-shuffle of the global power structure-which will be measured by new parameters and not just be limited to economic and military clout.

It remains undeniable that in the post-COVID scenario, the global challenges would be far more uncertain, ambiguous, volatile, unpredictable, and complex. This will cause the emerging world order to be marked by three key indicators: first, a further increase in technological innovation and advancement to maximise security; second, a greater competition among global powers, especially between the USA and China; and third, an increasing demand from the affected countries to identify and pin down 'the zoonotic source' of the virus and likewise, seek a response of the country of origin and address the failings of the WHO. These indicators are likely to result in greater polarisation among countries, based on their alignments and national interests- with 'national security' at the apex.

Recommendations: *Seeking a Way Forward from the Crisis*

Historically, every adversity has resulted in enhanced innovations and unique ideas to seize opportunities in emerging situations. Howard Gardener's seminal book, *Five Minds for the Future*, suggests that 'mind' should create solutions to new problems, questions, and phenomena.[33] Upholding this perception, the COVID-19 pandemic provides India with a timely opportunity to transform its old traditional ways of thinking and into novel methods and technology-centric approach to its national security. This monumental health, economic and psychological challenge should be converted into opportunities in myriad fields. Based on the experience gained, besides giving further impetus to the '*Swachch Bharat*' movement, we should see the emergence of a more robust and cooperative relationship between the Centre and the States. While some actions are already at hand by the government, the key suggestions are:

I. Health Care and Technology-Enabled Systems

Traditionally, health care has remained a low priority in India when seen in terms of allocation of budget, number of hospitals, polyclinics, medical facilities, doctors-to-population ratio, per capita hospital beds, health insurance, etc. Therefore, the aim should be:

- To prevent further spread of COVID-19 and provide adequate healthcare to save lives of people affected by it. It must plan to invest in healthcare facilities, protective measures, isolation facilities, drug and vaccine development programmes, R&D, training of staff, and infrastructure to minimise effects of such infectious diseases. To be responsive and innovative, the broad guidelines should flow out of a central authority and thereafter it should be delegated to state and local authorities to implement an action plan based on central guidelines and actual conditions existing on the ground.
- In an epidemic/pandemic, the management strategy should revolve around availability of 'comprehensive database of the country's population', use of technology-based systems to identify and track contacts, and monitor social distancing, provide an effective system of communicating policies and guidelines, and ruthless implementation. Progressively, India should work towards it.

- COVID-19 Is likely to persist for long, which is evident from emergence of second wave of the pandemic. The efforts to find medical solution and vaccines require concerted efforts to bring the pandemic under control. Concurrently, special medical schemes, health insurance policies, and guidelines to private hospitals regarding treatment and cost should be introduced to handle infectious diseases such as COVID-19.

II. Building Economy with Focus on Implementation on the Ground

It remains indisputable that having a 'strong economy' is one of the most powerful weapons in the world. However, to be a strong economy, sustained economic growth should be the highest priority of the country. This will help address the legitimate political, economic, social, and environmental requirements and the aspirations of the people, as also provide security and stability to them. In addition, a strong economy also requires providing security from NTS threats like water, food, health, energy, cyber, environmental degradation, and biological agents and infectious diseases like SARS, MERS-CoV and COVID-19. A 20 Lakh Crore Rupees 'stimulus package' has already been announced as a recovery measure. However, the major challenge lies in creating demand and immediate circulation of money to reboot the economy given the weaknesses related to the existing structural, regulatory and taxation systems, lack of physical and technological infrastructures, and long drawn bureaucratic procedures. Thereby, to build a sustained economy, India needs to be 'competitive' with its peers; and thus, need to adopt the following measures:

- Besides structural reforms, revival of economy will take place by strengthening start-ups, banking reforms, entrepreneurs, creating demand, reviewing of restrictive laws on labour, export, licensing, competitive corporate tax regime, excessive governance that is stifling enterprise and growth etc. However, 'implementation on the ground' should be central to India's economic strategy.
- The concept of 'Special Economic Zones' (SEZs) needs to be further incentivised, by giving priority loans, tax exemptions, tax holidays, according time bound approvals with minimal bureaucratic hurdles to encourage industries from investing in

select fields. A revised policy on SEZs needs to be formulated on an urgent basis.

- India must plan to emerge as a leading global player in sectors such as pharmaceuticals, IT, defence equipment, automobiles, cyber security, agricultural implements, engineering goods, and other products.
- Reforms be carried out to facilitate ease of doing business for multi-national companies that plan to shift their industries and businesses to India. The Micro, Small and Medium Enterprises (MSMEs) sector, which is the key driver of the Indian economy contributing 45 percent of total industrial production and 37.54 per cent of India's GDP,[34] should be revived by the government by innovative means. Israel is an excellent example which has given a boost to its start-ups to even make inroads into the Israeli Defence Ecosystem.
- While navigating the COVID crisis, multiple opportunities would be available to the business houses. They need to revisit their work cultures, requirement of technology related infrastructure, risks and safety mechanisms, talent retention and collaborations, importance of employees and customers, increased cyber threats in digital world, working together with the government, and others.
- 'Make in India' must be monitored continuously. Due attention should be given to the agricultural, and fishing sectors which employs around 70 per cent of India's working population, by way of pricing of their products and additional incentives.
- A wholistic view of the strengths and vulnerabilities of supply chains of essential commodities and items is imperative. India should adopt more open and welcoming policies and reduce tariffs, to facilitate Indian companies become a part of the 'global supply chain'. Simultaneously, e-Commerce should be given the necessary impetus to enhance India's economy.
- The government must work towards overcoming the vulnerabilities in India's informal sector that stood exposed especially after the outbreak of the pandemic.
- The government needs to analyse whether large-scale migration from urban to rural areas due to COVID-19 could cause any

long-term challenge or will it remain limited to the short-term challenge of 'shortage of labour'.

III. Proactive Foreign Policy

India needs to review its diplomatic relations and engage in developing close relations with its immediate and extended neighbourhood. In doing so, India needs to adopt the following measures:

- With the pandemic resulting into a softening of relations between a few Arab countries and Iran, India should utilise this opportunity to further enhance its relations with the region.
- With the likely changes in the strategic environment in Asia, IOR and the Indo-Pacific region, India should aim to diversify its trade relations as well as developing defence cooperation and/or strategic partnership with like-minded global powers, and a select number of other countries. By improving its capabilities in the IOR, India should emerge as the 'Net Security Provider and First Responder to Disasters'.
- India should maintain a close watch on the developments in the South China Sea to further enhance its relations with countries in South East Asia.
- India should boost its diplomatic outreach and assistance in fighting the pandemic in needy countries. COVID-19 provides huge potential to India to explore medical diplomacy, as it offers opportunities in the realm of domestic stability, economic cum commercial ventures, and strategic engagement with friendly foreign countries. Committed medical and pharmaceutical support to countries in need can be leveraged to improve India's diplomatic relations. Thereby, it must be pursued to win friends and to enter strategic partnerships.

IV. Defence Preparedness

Given the envisaged threats to our national security, both external and internal, the defence forces must not compromise on 'force preservation and battle readiness'. The measures to be taken are:

- In the short-term, each service should carry out innovative methods to optimise its resources, both in the short-term and long-term perspectives. A review of the existing systems, procedures, training, exercises, human resource management, rationalisation of manpower, ceremonial and administrative needs, capital works, new raisings and equipment, indigenisation, new technologies, etc., would throw up some solutions. Battle readiness should not be compromised at any cost.

- As the Defence Cyber & Space Agencies and Special Operations Division are niche capabilities at strategic-operational levels, these must be developed, as planned. There is a need to develop indigenous capabilities to create redundancies; thus, securing India's operational readiness through self-reliance.
- The pertinent question is whether Defence Research and Development Organisation (DRDO) will be able to provide the 'cutting edge technologies in select fields' to our armed forces? It is time that DRDO and private home-grown organisations should work with a mission-oriented zeal to deliver such indigenously built technologies and networks to enhance the reliability and security architecture.
- Simultaneously, seize the opportunity to carry out structural reforms and transformation of India's Defence Industrial Base (DIB) and DRDO by taking certain hard decisions. Finally, the aim should be to graduate to an 'export-oriented industry'.
- In the long-term perspective, India needs to develop its infrastructure on the borders, and the defence forces must progressively build soft, hard, and demonstrated military power to deter threats to its stability and integrity. A strong military muscle deters an adversary to pose threats while combating a pandemic. A case in point is China's transgressions across the LAC in the midst of COVID-19 in May- June 2020. Given China's aggressive behaviour at the LAC in Eastern Ladakh, it is an excellent lesson for the Indian Armed Forces to maintain a balanced military posture, upgrade its intelligence and surveillance capabilities, remain vigilant, and be battle ready against deceitful adversaries even during pandemics. Integration and jointness is the way forward to ensure timely decisions and synergised actions against adversaries.
- Along with the pressures of military operations, a country's

security will also be adversely affected if its population is subjected to information warfare campaigns[35]—as caused by persistent perception management, propaganda, and psychological narratives propagated by its adversaries. India must take a note of such simultaneous actions by its adversaries, and formulate a media policy at the national level.

- With growing isolation of China due to the aftereffects of COVID-19, there is a possibility of greater military integration between China and Pakistan. This nexus could then keep India engaged at both fronts over a wide spectrum of conflicts.

V. IT Industry, Digital Revolution and Virtual Interactions

India has an advantage of a strong mix of young and technically trained professionals, especially from institutes such as IITs and IIMs that bring out professional talent with diverse skills. It must lead the world in inventing new ways and platforms that support the new social norms of working from home, virtual interactions, educational systems, and digital transactions. The Digital Revolution has transformed our society, as it has affected every facet of our daily lives: retail, banking, e-commerce, business, healthcare, defence systems, travel and tourism, education, and entertainment. New mechanisms such as work from home, virtual interactions and meetings should be adopted to enhance efficiency and keep the work force operational. The 'Digital India' campaign requires a further impetus to reach out to every village and citizen. Post COVID-19, digitalisation has been one of the fundamental examples of 'frugal innovation and implementation' the world over.

VI. Education and Technology

It is the need of the hour that every village and town in India should be digitally connected for better interaction, both to further education as well as connectivity. Fundamental structural changes should be made in the curriculum/syllabi/programmes to attract students from across the country. It should be noted that higher education and technology are crucial factors in improving national prosperity. Progressively, we should provide low cost digital devices to students across the country, and graduate to live virtual educational classrooms and examinations. Skill development should be part of the curriculum in engineering and science degree programmes. This will create future entrepreneurs, create employment opportunities, and further enhance the business skills amongst Indian youth.

VII. Migrant Work Force Ministry

While the national lockdown has certainly delayed the casualties and has flattened the curve, it has caused an unprecedented loss both in terms of life and livelihood on India's overwhelming migrant labour population. Although a Union Labour Ministry is in place, but the current situation calls for the need to create a separate Migrant Work Force Ministry at the Centre, with related departments in each state, to maintain the data and meet the aspirations of over 120 million migrant work force within the country and abroad. This has also highlighted the need for a comprehensive review of the public distribution system (PDS) to cater for such emergencies.

VIII. Employment Opportunities

According to CMIE, the rate of unemployment had increased to 24 per cent on 17 May 2020 (the figures are likely to be more than as highlighted given the informal sector has been affected the most). Being a demographically young country, all elements of national power should work innovatively to provide challenging job opportunities to its youth—a high priority responsibility.

IX. Environmental Security

As environmental degradation (air pollution, water pollution etc,) is intricately linked to the health index of a country, the country needs to promote awareness, allocate adequate budget, and focus on preventing the adverse effects of it on priority. Stricter laws on industrial and medical waste management must be formulated and implemented.

X. Internal Security and Societal Harmony

Due to slow down in economy, return of migrant work force to rural areas, sharp increase in unemployment rate and affected people finding difficult to get essential needs, insurgents, especially in Maoists' affected areas in Central India, are likely to recruit cadres into their fold. The returning migrants and their families should be provided necessary help, jobs to prevent exploitation of hapless people by the insurgents. The current pandemic crisis is an excellent opportunity to resolve some of India's insurgencies by engaging with the insurgents, fulfilling some of their legitimate aspirations, and survival needs. It requires a mission-oriented approach to achieve it.

Here, the aim must be to fight the virus and the life-threatening diseases, and not allow issues to turn to a law and order situation due to irresponsible statements by leaders and reporting by the media. Every citizen and leader must be respectful towards the sensitivities of each religion, region, caste, and ethnic community, to maintain the 'integrity and secular fabric' of the country. Suitable laws be enacted to prevent and deter such incidents.

XI. Information Dissemination System

Due to fake news, misinformation, and lack of a timely correct information in the environment, it resulted in the severity of the humanitarian crisis. With panic predominant mainly among the migrant workers and poor people, it is an important lesson to learn and demands to be corrected immediately by formulating a policy on strategic communication and media.

Conclusion

Given the severity of COVID-19, it should be India's endeavour to exploit the opportunities by acting with a sense of urgency. Here, one of the most important objectives for the government would be to take care of the sick and prevent further spread of the pandemic; re-boot the economy (survive, revive, and grow); provide support to industries, agriculture, MSMEs, mining, infrastructure and construction; create job opportunities; and adopt structural reforms to simplify and improve the efficiency of the system. To seize the opportunities created by the current crisis, India needs to adopt a technology-centric approach to identify focus areas and act simultaneously on several fronts as part of its national strategy. Furthermore, India should synergise the strengths of all the available elements of its national power, not just the military alone, to make India 'Future Ready', especially post COVID-19.

NOTES

1 SARS, the first global epidemic in the 21st century, affected 26 countries and resulted in more than 8,000 cases in 2003. For details see World Health Organization, "SARS (Severe Acute Respiratory Syndrome)", https://www.who.int/ith/diseases/sars/en/, accessed online 14 May 2020.

2 Since 2012, 27 countries have reported cases of MERS. For details see World Health Organization, "Middle East respiratory syndrome coronavirus (MERS-CoV)", 11 May 2019, https://www.who.int/news-room/fact-sheets/detail/middle-east-respiratory-syndrome-coronavirus-(mers-cov), accessed online 14 May 2020.

3 Richard P. Wenzel et al. (2005), "Lessons from Severe Acute Respiratory Syndrome (SARS): Implications for Infection Control", *Arch Med Res.*, vol. 36, no. 6, pp. 610–616.

4 Stockholm International Peace Research Institute (2020), "Global military expenditure sees largest annual increase in a decade-says SIPRI-reaching $1917 billion in 2019", 27 April 2020, https://www.sipri.org/research/armament-and-disarmament/arms-and-military-expenditure/military-expenditure, accessed online 15 May 2020.

5 See, World Health Organization, "WHO Coronavirus Disease (COVID-19) Dashboard", https://covid19.who.int/, accessed online 30 June 2020.

6 Ibid.

7 See "Coronavirus Worldwide Graphs", *Worldometer*, https://www.worldometers.info/coronavirus/worldwide-graphs/#total-cases, accessed online 30 June 2020.

8 See *Worldometer*, https://www.worldometers.info/coronavirus/country/india/, accessed online 30 June 2020.

9 United Nations Development Programme (1994), *Human Development* Report, New York: Oxford University Press, pp. 22-46, http://www.hdr.undp.org/sites/default/files/reports/255/hdr_1994_en_complete_nostats.pdf, accessed online 16 May 2020.

10 Ibid., p. 23.

11 National interests include national identity, sovereignty, territorial integrity; security of state, society and people, preservation of the institutions, sustainable economic development, secure environment for people, human security from non-traditional security threats, and retain pride in one's history, language, culture, heritage, customs and traditions and others.

12 See, NTS-Asia, "About Non-Traditional Security", https://rsis-ntsasia.org/about-nts-asia/, accessed online 16 May 2020.

13 Saurabh Chaudhuri, "Defining Non-Traditional Security Threats", *Global India Foundation*, https://www.globalindiafoundation.org/nontraditionalsecurity.html, accessed online 15 May 2020.

14 See, NTS-Asia, "About Non-Traditional Security", n. 12.

15 Saurabh Chaudhuri, "Defining Non-Traditional Security Threats", n. 13.

16 See NTS-Asia, "About Non-Traditional security", n. 12.

17 United Nations Development Programme (1994), *Human Development* Report, n. 9.

18 World Health Organization (2018), "Managing Epidemics: Key Facts About Managing Epidemics", Version 1, p. 22, https://www.who.int/emergencies/diseases/managing-epidemics-interactive.pdf, accessed online 14 May 2020.

19 Yizhou Wang (2004), "Defining Non-Traditional Security and Its Implications for China," *China & World Economy*, vol. 12, p. 63.

20 Douglas Broom (2020), "6 of the world's 10 most polluted cities are in India," *World Economic Forum*, 05 March 2020, https://www.weforum.org/agenda/2020/03/6-of-the-world-s-10-most-polluted-cities-are-in-india/, accessed on 20 May 2020.

21 Satya Priya and Aidan Cronin, "UN report on "Water in India: Situation and prospects" rings alarm on water scarcity in the country," *Indiawaterportal*, https://www.indiawaterportal.org/news/un-report-water-india-situation-and-prospects-rings-alarm-water-scarcity-country, accessed online 30 May 2020.

22 See Ministry of Environment, Forests and Climate Change, Demand No. 25, p. 84, https://www.indiabudget.gov.in/doc/eb/sbe25.pdf,accessed online 20 May 2020.

23 Among the biggest employers of migrant workers is the construction sector (40 million), domestic work (20 million), textile (11 million), brick kiln work (10 million), transportation, mines & quarries, and agriculture. As per official figures of India Labour Migration Update 2018, there are over 30 million Indians overseas. See "Labour and Migration in India," *Ajeevika Bureau*, http://www.aajeevika.org/labour-and-migration.php, accessed online 28 May 2020.

24 According to India's 2011 Census data, the slum population as percentage of city's population are: Greater Mumbai (8.3 mn or 41.3 per cent, Kolkata (2 mn or 29.6 per cent), Chennai (2 mn or 28.5 per cent), Delhi (2.9 mn or 14.6 per cent).

25 Puja Mehra (2020), "India's economy needs big dose of health spending, *Live Mint*, 08 April 2020, https://www.livemint.com/news/india/india-s-economy-needs-big-dose-of-health-spending-11586365603651.html, accessed online 18 May 2020.

26 Ibid.

27 Michael Beckley (2019), "The US should fear a Faltering China," *Foreign Affairs*, 28 October 2019, https://www.foreignaffairs.com/articles/china/2019-10-28/united-states-should-fear-faltering-china, accessed online 17 May 2020.

28 See International Monetary Fund (2020), "World Economic Outlook Update", June 2020, https://www.imf.org/en/Publications/WEO/Issues/2020/06/24/WEOUpdateJune2020, accessed online 24 June 2020.

29 Ibid.

30 Ibid.

31 See International Monetary Fund (2020), "World Economic Outlook Update", n. 28.

32 See Centre for Monitoring Indian Economy Pvt Ltd (2020), "Hard Times Ahead," 19 May 2020, https://www.cmie.com/kommon/bin/sr.php?kall=warticle&dt=2020-05-19%2008:41:03&msec=086, accessed online 30 May 2020.

33 See Howard Gardner (2006), *Five Minds for the Future*, Boston, MA: Harvard Business Review Press.

34 MSME Policy, "Launch of Draft Consultation Paper", https://msme.gov.in/sites/default/files/MSME%20Policy%20final%20document.pdf, accessed online 23 June 2020.

35 China has aggressively followed its Three Warfare Strategy (2010) of media warfare, psychological warfare and legal warfare to influence perceptions of its domestic population and global community.

2

India's Alarming Call: Need for Greater Sustainability

Manjari Singh

With the world facing an unprecedented challenge of the COVID-19 pandemic there is a growing realisation towards adapting to the "new normal".[1] Thomas Friedman, noted opinion journalist with the *New York Times* and winner of the Pulitzer Prize, remarked that amongst all the disparities and divisions existing in the world, the most strikingly notable one would be the new historical division of the world Before Corona (B.C.) and After Corona (A.C.).[2] Given the number of years it takes for a stark shift to take place, Friedman equated the change with Before Christ (B.C.) and *Anno Domini* (A.D.). Needless to mention, that the changing dynamics call for re-defining various age-old concepts and ideas including a re-thinking on what corresponds to national interests. While the new virus has highlighted the inter-connectivity of today's world, the ways in which national, regional and international actors have responded to the crisis in their respective countries reveals their readiness in the face of future emerging challenges.

In the Indian context, the first-aid response to declaration of countrywide lockdown on 24 March was not only a smart decision but suggests that the decision makers were closely observing the COVID-19 surge globally. However, in the midst of preparations for a lockdown, India was caught off-guard especially with regard to making arrangements for the marginal sections of society. Keeping the house in order at such short notice and that too when India has a huge population density and size, topped with many other complexities, is a Herculean task. The bigger question, however, is what next?

While the short-term implications are being realised with the mayhem that has been created, slowing of economy, increase in unemployment rate, problems in education system, inability to deal with other health issues, shortage of medical equipment, food crisis especially for the marginal sections of society, and others- are calling for a massive need for preparedness in the mid-term and long-term A.C. situation.

As is evident, there has been a dramatic shift in the perception of what encompasses the securing of 'national interests', which is mainly defined as a survival strategy that is achieved by the "protection of physical, political, and cultural identity against encroachments by other nation-states".[3] However, the present context of COVID-19 demands the need to expand the type, nature and form of 'encroachment' as the world today is fighting a 'faceless enemy' in the form of a virus. This has changed the security dynamics from the traditional notion of protecting the territorial borders to that of taking an inclusive approach towards national security that involves both traditional and non-traditional security considerations. This makes the economic, social, and environmental factors as equally important to the political and military ones. However, it seems A.C., the former will overshadow the latter in the coming future.[4] When and how it will happen still remains uncertain.

What is noteworthy is that COVID-19 has forced social scientists to call for the imminent need for a reorientation to the age-old concepts, international agencies, value systems, state priorities and others, which stand invalid and redundant in the present context. Notwithstanding traditional security issues, a pandemic such as COVID-19 has made the world realise its ill-preparedness when it comes to handling a non-traditional threat of such high magnitude. Notably, despite many warnings by noted climatologists and agencies such as Intergovernmental Panel on Climate Change (IPCC) about the threats posed by climate change and the resultant increase in pandemics, the states were not ready to focus their policies towards human, social and environmental securities.[5] With the global economy projected to contract sharply by 3 per cent in 2020[6] and projected global unemployment rate standing at 32.1 percent,[7] COVID-19 has called for a reality check on the growing insecurities related to heath, food, income disparities and many more.

The changing dynamics require India to adopt a sustainable approach in its national policy under the changing security situation. For, with few protectionist measures in place, nations are trying to 'save their own' first. In this perspective, this chapter argues that these can be done by giving the sustainable development approach its due and long-awaited credit. While India's performance prior to the pandemic was poor, especially in the hunger and poverty fields, a fresh approach to it is essential which will require a detailed analysis of the short-term and long-term impact of COVID-19.

Sustainable Development: *Integral to Rescue National Interests*

Awareness of the sustainable development aspect of national security the world over is a recent phenomenon. The modernisation paradigm of the 1950s focused solely on hard core developmental aspects of economic growth and it was only in the 1980s, three decades later, when the need to sustain development was felt by conserving the environment.[8] Defined in 1987 by the UN-mandated Brundtland Commission, sustainable development means "one that meets the needs of the present without compromising the ability of future generations to meet their own needs".[9]

This means that there are three significant components highlighted in the definition: "a desirable human condition, an enduring ecosystem, and a balance between the present and future generations".[10] However, it is important to note that it took almost another three decades (about 28 years) for the UN to chart out 17 comprehensive sustainable development goals (SDGs) in January 2015 (See Figure 2.1). In a pilot project form, Millennium Development Goals (MDGs) of 2000-2015 for each country, served as the building blocks for SDGs.

Figure 2.1: Seventeen Sustainable Development Goals

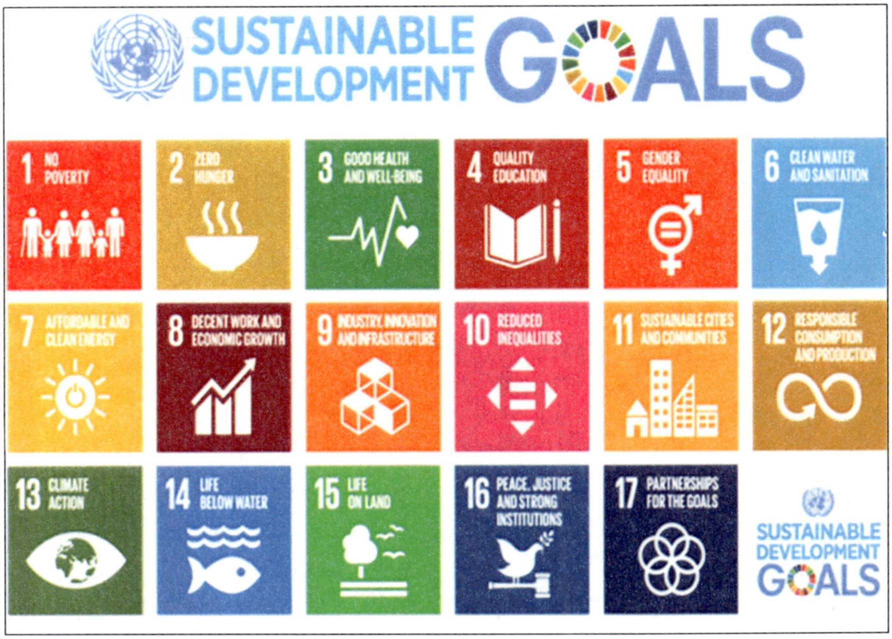
SUSTAINABLE DEVELOPMENT GOALS
1 NO POVERTY
2 ZERO HUNGER
3 GOOD HEALTH AND WELL-BEING
4 QUALITY EDUCATION
5 GENDER EQUALITY
6 CLEAN WATER AND SANITATION
7 AFFORDABLE AND CLEAN ENERGY
8 DECENT WORK AND ECONOMIC GROWTH
9 INDUSTRY, INNOVATION AND INFRASTRUCTURE
10 REDUCED INEQUALITIES
11 SUSTAINABLE CITIES AND COMMUNITIES
12 RESPONSIBLE CONSUMPTION AND PRODUCTION
13 CLIMATE ACTION
14 LIFE BELOW WATER
15 LIFE ON LAND
16 PEACE, JUSTICE AND STRONG INSTITUTIONS
17 PARTNERSHIPS FOR THE GOALS
SUSTAINABLE DEVELOPMENT GOALS

Source: UNDESA, 2017.[11]

Ranging from "no poverty" and "zero hunger" to "peace, justice and strong institutions", SDGs are inclusive of all the sectors of development, namely, social, economic, environmental and political. To achieve these goals, United Nations Department for Economic and Social Affairs (UN DESA) urged the UN signatories to set their timers to 2025 or 2030 to achieve these goals as part of its *Visions*.

In the South Asian context which has enormous population pressure and majority of the countries being developing economies; non-traditional challenges including poverty, hunger, malnutrition and others have become critical not only to their economic welfare but also for political stability. Keeping this in mind, sustainable development has been viewed as a holistic concept, which aims at a more comprehensive development; that is, of the society, economy and environment.

However, challenges to sustainable development in South Asia hovers around achieving "No Poverty" and "Zero Hunger" The World

Bank defines the International Poverty Line at US$ 1.9 per capita but more than a fifth of the population of South Asia or over 350 million people live below this level and out of this 13.5 per cent are identified as living in extreme poverty. Similarly, in terms of hunger, 15.7 per cent of the global undernourished population or more than 280 million live in South Asia.

In short, nearly a fifth of the South Asian population lives under extreme poverty and hungry despite the region being predominantly an agrarian economy.[12] When it comes to India, it fares extremely low in these two indicators. It is ranked 102 out of 117 countries in the global hunger index (GHI) in 2019 (lower than Pakistan, Nepal, Bangladesh and Sri Lanka).[13] During the same time in 2019, India ranked 49th on the Poverty Index and it was found out that more than 36 crore Indians cannot afford a decent three square meals a day.[14] Therefore, achieving SDGs becomes crucial for India to safeguard its national interests; however, there are many challenges facing it.

SDGs: *India's Ground Realities*

India adopted SDGs in September 2015 as part of a resolution, "Transforming our world: the 2030 agenda for sustainable development". The onus lies on the NITI Aayog to "bring together stakeholders and build capacities for the realization of SDGs" and thus, the organisation "has organized several national and regional level consultations".[15] While the NITI Aayog has brought out a few points on "achievements in the year 2018-19," the actual results seem to be at a low and still in the infant stage. Moreover, the 181-page report released by the NITI Aayog in December 2019 and titled *SDG India: Index and Dashboard 2019-20*, gives merely state and UT level geographical distribution on each indicator in SDGs. It lacks depth and analysis and has a skewed approach of understanding the subject. The real picture can only be revealed at unit level analysis.

In 2019, India ranked 115 out of 162 countries on the SDG Index with a score of 61.1 and is behind a few South Asian neighbours such as Maldives (47), Bhutan (84), Sri Lanka (93) and Nepal (103). The rest of the South Asian nations like Bangladesh (116), Pakistan (130), and Afghanistan (153) are the only ones that rank lower than India.[16] This suggests that even before the outbreak of the pandemic, India was not developing sustainably. In fact, until the arrival of the new virus, the country had just started to realise the importance of the concept and was busy collecting data on various aspects of development. The NITI Aayog formulated methodologies to collect data at the state and UT levels on the 17 SDGs; however, the changing dynamics calls for a fresh look at the subject. Moreover, while the ranking suggests that India lags behind in almost all the social, economic and environmental dimensions (See Figure 2.2), SDG 1 and SDG 2 are of critical concern to New Delhi (See Figures 2.3 and Figure 2.4).

While the overall ranking of the country is not very promising, the geographical distribution of SDGs gives an idea as to which states need more attention. Figure 2.2 denotes that only the southern states of the country, Sikkim and Himachal Pradesh, are "front runners" in achieving the SDGs (score ranges between 65-99), the rest of the states and UTs are merely "performers" with a score range of 50-64. It is saddening to see that none is an "achiever". It is to be noted that going further deep to the unit and municipality levels, the situation will be grimmer and the stark differences will be noticeable.

India fares extremely low on SDG 1 with a global ranking of 102 out of 117 countries on GHI in 2019. A report published by the NITI Aayog in December 2019 reveals that while Tamil Nadu and Jammu and Kashmir are the top performing State and Union Territory respectively, six states including Tripura, Andhra Pradesh, Meghalaya, Mizoram, Sikkim and Kerala are "front runners" with scores higher than 65. However, there are about 14 states and three UTs that fall behind in the aspirant category (See Figure 2.3). The report further suggests that some improvement is made in the field by reduction of the poverty rate to 21.92 per cent of the Indian population, which lives below the poverty line.

Figure 2.4 shows the performance of Indian states and UTs on the hunger index. According to the NITI Aayog, in 2019 around 20 states and three UTs scored less than 50 out of 100 in the "Zero hunger" category. This is an alarming situation as only seven states

Figure 2.2: India's Performance in 17 SDGs

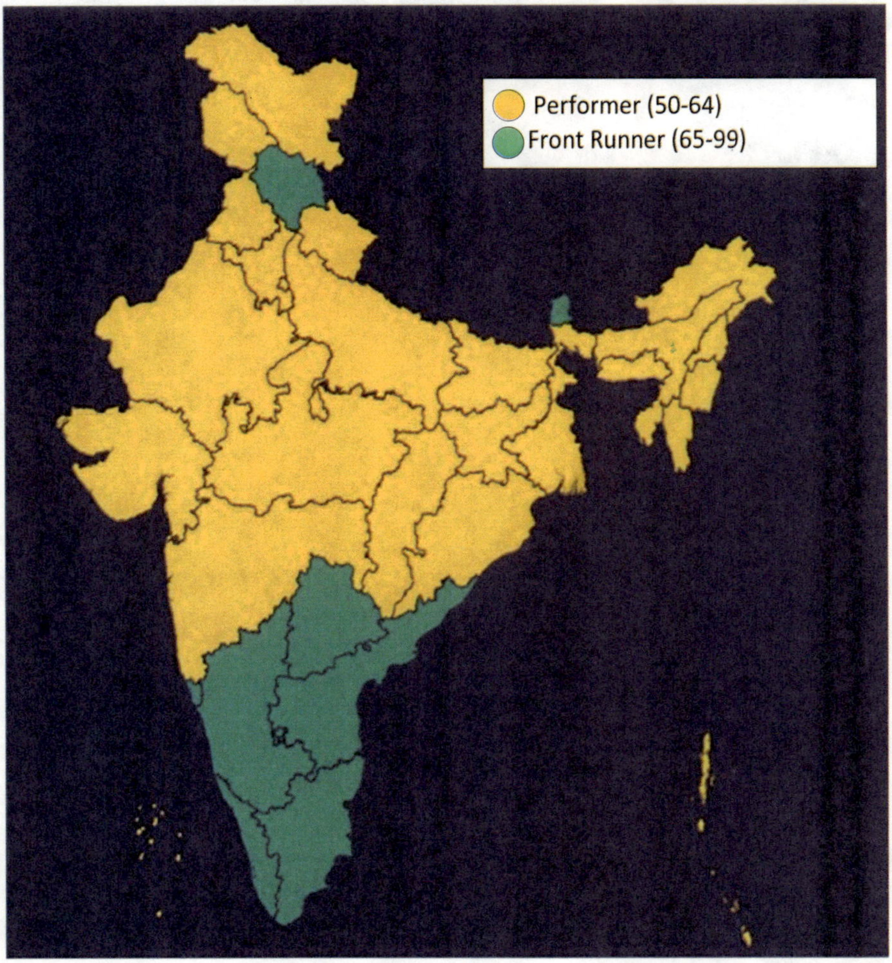

Source: Adapted from UN-NITI Aayog, 2019.[17]

Figure 2.3: India's Performance (State-wise) on SDG 1, "No Poverty"

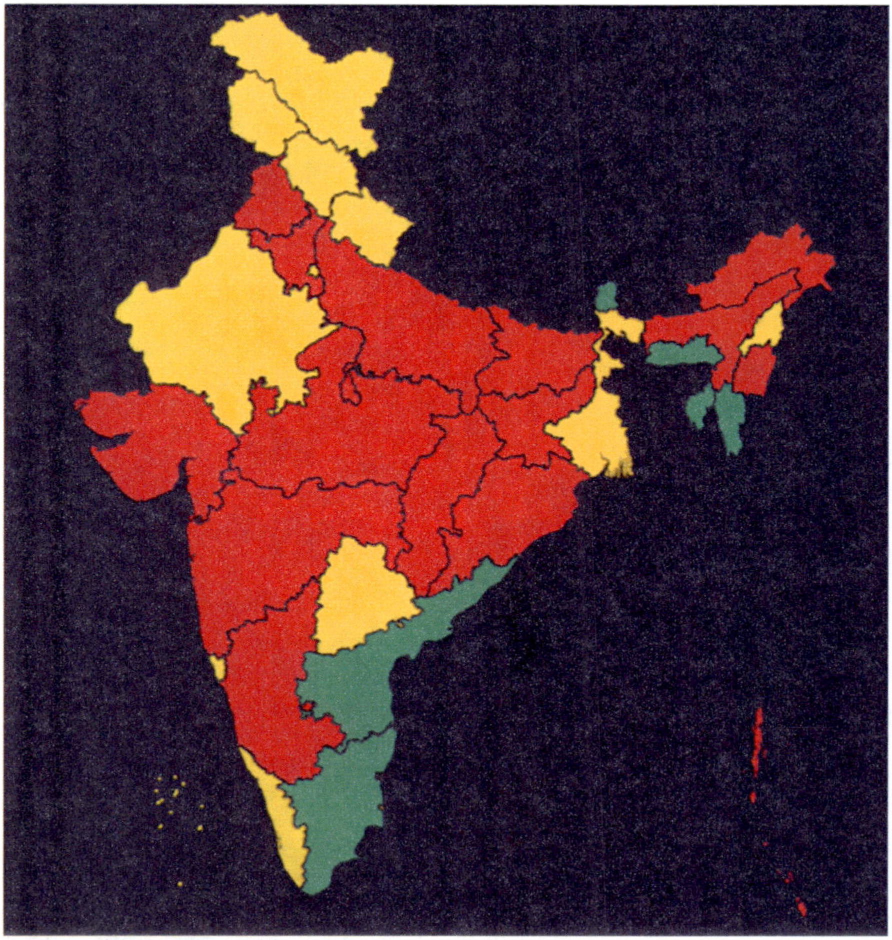

Aspirant (0-49)
Chhattisgarh, Karnataka, Assam, Punjab, Gujarat, Haryana, Maharashtra, Odisha, Manipur, Madhya Pradesh, Uttar Pradesh, Arunachal Pradesh, Bihar, Jharkhand, Andaman & Nicobar Islands, Chandigarh, Dadra & Nagar Haveli

Performer (50-64)
Kerala, Uttarakhand, Himachal Pradesh, Nagaland, Rajasthan, Goa, Telangana, West Bengal, Daman & Diu, Jammu & Kashmir, Ladakh, Lakshadweep, Puducherry, Delhi

Front Runner (65-99)
Tamil Nadu, Tripura, Andhra Pradesh, Meghalaya, Mizoram, Sikkim

Achiever (100)

Source: Adapted from UN-NITI Aayog, 2019.[18]

Figure 2.4: India's Performance on SDG 2, "Zero Hunger"

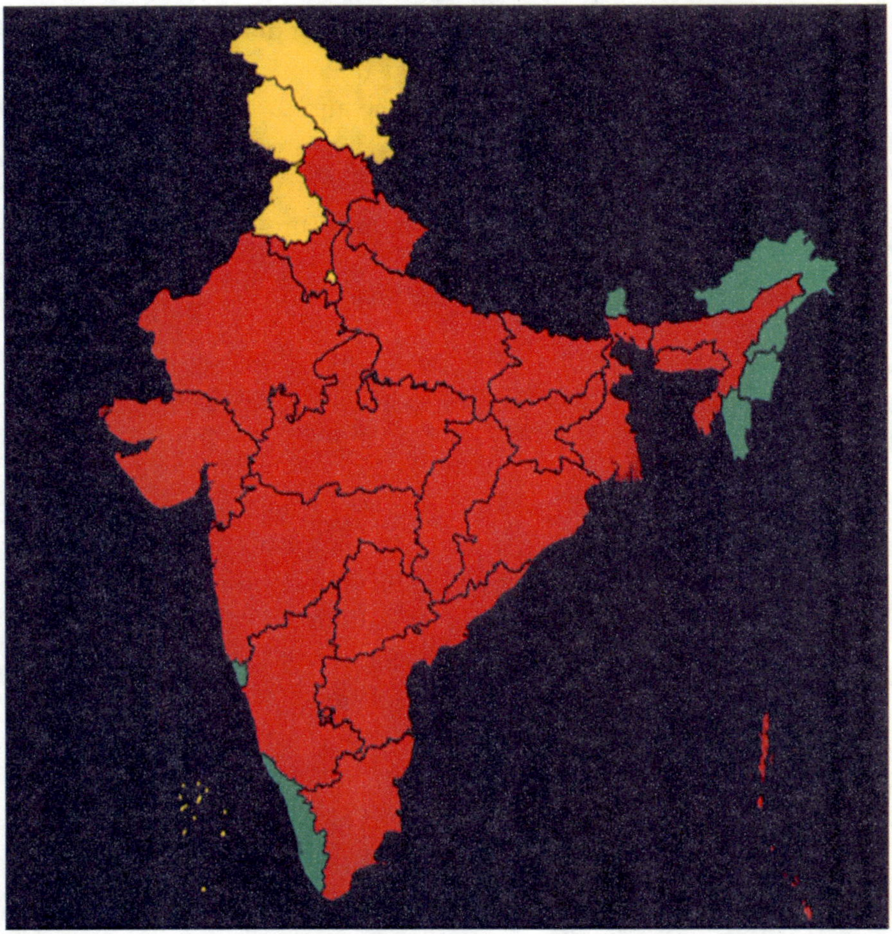

Aspirant (0-49)
Tripura, Tamil Nadu, Uttarakhand, Himachal Pradesh, Haryana, West Bengal, Assam, Gujarat, Karnataka, Telangana, Andhra Pradesh, Meghalaya, Rajasthan, Maharashtra, Odisha, Uttar Pradesh, Chhattisgarh, Bihar, Madhya Pradesh, Jharkhand, Dadra & Nagar Haveli, Andaman & Nicobar Islands, Daman & Diu

Performer (50-64)
Punjab, Lakshadweep, Delhi, Jammu & Kashmir, Ladakh

Front Runner (65-99)
Mizoram, Kerala, Nagaland, Manipur, Arunachal Pradesh, Sikkim, Chandigarh, Puducherry

Achiever (100)

Source: Adapted from UN-NITI Aayog, 2019.[19]

and two UTs fared better on the indicator and are "front runners".[20] Nearly 33.4 per cent of children in India are underweight as per NITI Aayog statistics. The report mentioned that 34.7 per cent of children under the age of five are stunted and the aim through the report was to reduce this to 2.5 per cent by 2030. This already seemed to be an over-ambitious goal to achieve in merely 11 years; however, post-pandemic will result in more children in future being malnourished and stunted.

While hunger and poverty percentages are likely to increase after the advent of the coronavirus pandemic, there is a window of opportunity too, that if managed well, can help India in containing these indicators and will have a multiplier effect on the economy in the long run. India being an agrarian economy, and largest employment generator in the country, produced 2,516.67 kg of rice, wheat, and coarse cereals per hectare of land annually prior to the outbreak of the virus.[21] The plan was to double the produce by 2030, and that probably can be achieved. With most of the migrant labour back in their villages, agriculture will serve as the saviour as there is the least probability that these workers will go back to cities and towns to their old jobs, and thus more focus can be attributed to boosting agricultural productivity. However, this will require well-structured planning.

While India performs badly on the two indicators mentioned above, gender inequality remains a growing challenge for the country. However, the 2019 NITI Aayog report revealed that on other indicators or goals, India's performance was noticeable, but again state and UT-level statistics will only result in a skewed understanding of the situation in the country. Economic growth leading to decent work forms a crucial component in achieving SDGs but interestingly, before the onset of the pandemic followed by nationwide lockdowns, India's economic growth rate had fallen and the economic performance was rather low at a 11-year low of 5 per cent.[22]

On the environmental sustainability front, India did not do any better during pre-COVID-19 times. Pollution in big cities and metros, poor management of waste, growing water scarcity especially in remote areas, poor air quality, biodiversity loss, land degradation, climate change, etc., have been major concerns in India.[23] Nevertheless, the advent of coronavirus in India had a ripple effect over the looming challenges already facing India, especially in two dimensions—economic and social. This makes it imperative to venture into understanding the immediate impact of COVID-19 and, thereafter, assess the long-term impacts on sustainability as a result of the coronavirus.

Impact of COVID-19: *Taking Stock of Social and Economic Sustainability in India*

A global snapshot suggests that a recession as brutal as during the Great Depression is approaching post-pandemic. The extent is expected to be so vast that the IMF has called it "the Great Lockdown".[24] Worldwide lockdowns are immediately adversely affecting the economies and societies and are becoming challenging on an everyday basis. While the immediate impact of the virus is of concern, long-term implications will be more brutal if the problems are not identified and fixed through proper planning and management. The impacts of COVID-19 are divided into short-term and long-term for better understanding as to how the pandemic is affecting sustainability in India.

I. Short-Term Impact

Released in December 2019, the NITI Aayog report *SDG India: Index and Dashboard 2019-20* touted as SDG India Index 2.0 revealed disturbing findings regarding the county's performance on each goal. Based on data available tat hat time, various projections were made to achieve India's *Vision 2030*; however, the pandemic washed off all the efforts. It not only tampered with the positive results achieved in fields such as education, health, water, etc., but further brought down the figures of fields wherein India required focussed attention, namely, growing poverty, rate of unemployment, food insecurity, economic growth, income inequality and others.[25] The negative effect on the latter can be seen in the short-term phase; that is, during the pandemic itself.

The coronavirus outbreak has transformed from a global pandemic to a global crisis of the present. Medical implications, shortages in equipment supplies, psychological fear, etc., notwithstanding, the new virus has adversely affected the society and economy of nations.

While lockdowns and social distancing have restricted movement of population, loss of jobs and means to livelihood has resulted in mass reverse-migration, that is, from cities to villages. This phenomenon is a common sight in India as the nationwide lockdown has impacted 40 million internal migrants according to a study conducted by the World Bank.[26] The same report highlights that around 50,000-60,000 people moved from urban centres to rural areas "within a span of few days".[27] To ease this migration, government in a slightly delayed response set up camps with basic provisions to provide shelter to the migrants.

If internal mass displacements were not enough, many Indians came back or were evacuated from foreign countries facing the worse form of pandemic in various streams until the first week of May. In Phase I alone of the pandemic, India planned and evacuated about 14,800 stranded Indians from over 13 countries by using three Navy warships and 64 flights. Indians stranded in the UAE, UK, Saudi Arabia, Philippines, Singapore, Bangladesh, Qatar, Bahrain, the USA, Oman, Kuwait, etc., were evacuated in May.[28] Most notable evacuations wherein more than 1,800 Indians were brought back to India during February-March was from China, Italy and Iran. India evacuated 723 Indians from China[29] in February, 263 from Italy,[30] and 890 from Iran,[31] during that time.

In all, around 513 flights have been used as on May end to bring back Indians from various parts of the world as per the *Vande Bharat Mission* of the Ministry of External Affairs (MEA).[32] While this is a commendable effort on the part of the government, it also suggests that this is the time when India should frame its stringent and rigorous evacuation policy so that it is not caught off guard. The pandemic highlighted India's lack of a stringent evacuation policy. To note, India has been involved in evacuation operations since 1960s as noted in Table 2.1, but has been caught off guard every single time. This reflects India's lack of preparedness to form a policy on evacuation.

Evacuation of its citizenry is a noble deed but this also suggests that not just the government exchequer was utilised to put things in place; but the already high unemployment rate is expected to rise further and likewise, the remittances that India receives from its overseas Indians will also be tremendously affected. Notably, India is the top recipient of

Table 2.1: India's Expatriate Evacuation Operations (1962-2020)

Year	*Country*	*Evacuees/Total NRIs*
1962-63	Mozambique	2,300/2,400
1963-64	Burma, South-East Asia	300,000/500,000
1968	Kenya	2,500/NA
September-November 1972	Uganda	5,000/NA
1980	**Iraq**	11,000/NA
January 1986	**Yemen**	800/3,000
August-October 1990	**Kuwait/Gulf**	170,000/200,000
May 1994	**Yemen**	1,700-7,000
October 1996	**UAE**	60,000/NA
March 2003	**Kuwait**	3,500/300,000
July 2006	**Lebanon**	2,300/12,000
June 2010	Kyrgyzstan	110/NA
January-February 2011	**Egypt**	700/3,600
February-March 2011	**Libya**	16,400/18,000
June-August 2011	**Yemen**	700-800/ NA
May-June 2014	Ukraine	1,000/NA
2014-2015	**Libya**	3,600/5,600
April 2015	**Yemen**	6,700/NA
April-June 2015	Nepal	5,188/NA
2015	**Iraq**	7,000/NA
March 2016	Belgium	242/NA
July 2016	**South Sudan**	153/700
February 2020 (ongoing)	Globally	>15,000

Source: *Prepared by the Author in consultation with the Ministry of External Affairs Website, and Constantino Xavier (2016).*[33] [The maximum evacuation operations have been conducted in the Middle Eastern and North African regions, apparently the most conflict prone regions, as highlighted in bold.]

remittances in the world which amounts to US$ 83.1 billion and accounts for 2.8 per cent of Indian GDP. Owing to the corona crisis, India's remittances are projected to fall by 23 per cent in 2020, which will amount to US$ 64 billion.[34]

According to the CMIE, around 27 million youth in the age group 20-30 years and 30 million people in their 30s lost their jobs amidst the nationwide lockdown by April.[35] By May, the total unemployment rate reached 24 per cent. However, with few industries opening up gradually, on a weekly average basis, about 3.5 per cent increase is felt in the labour participation rate but the uncertainty continues to prevail because of intermittent lockdowns as infected cases rise.[36] Long-term implications of job loss will be very high in the next few years.

The growing unemployment rate has affected marginalised sections of society the most who were mostly employed in informal sectors of economy. As per an International Labour Organization (ILO) estimate, around 400 million Indians are at the risk of sinking below the poverty line.[37] Moreover, according to a World Bank report, around 30 million internal migrants were affected by the lockdown, which also amounts to the same number of job losses that forced these migrants to head for their homes.[38] The Periodic Labour Force Survey (PLFS) paints that as around 90 per cent of the total workforce population is employed in the informal sector (419 million out of 465 million total workforce population), disturbance in this sector will adversely affect the overall economy of the country. Of this, around 80 per cent of the workforce is employed in urban centres. About 93 million informal workers are involved in five sectors (manufacturing; trade, hotel and restaurants, construction; transport, storage and communication; and financial business and real estate) in urban areas and these are the most affected sectors during lockdowns. This has led to job loss, poverty, reverse-migration, health crisis and food insecurity. Inter-dependency of one factor to another is rather noticeable during such times.[39]

When it comes to an impact on sectors of the economy, *Statista* estimates the maximum impact of the virus on a few major sectors such as financial, real estate, and professional services (-17.3 per cent), mining and quarrying (-14.7 per cent), electricity, gas, water supply and other utilities (-13.9 per cent), construction (-13.3 per cent), trade, hotels, transport, communication and broadcasting services (-9.7 per cent), overall Gross Value Added (-9.3 per cent), manufacturing (-6.3 per cent), agriculture, forestry and fishing (-1.3 per cent), and public administration, defence and other services (-0.4 per cent).[40]

As is noted from the figure, the picture is not so grim for the agricultural and allied sectors. As per the NITI Aayog's assessment in April, "the farm sector is poised to grow" by 3 per cent despite disruption in the economy and remains to be the "beacon of hope" amidst the crisis due to COVID-19. With larger summer crop area than last year, higher sales of fertilizers and seeds and better prices, the sector has flourished. There has been an increase of 37 per cent in rice plantation areas. All of this has resulted in an increase of food production in the country by 3.7 per cent.[41] However, much needs to be done in order to provide advanced technologies, fertilisers and capital to the farmers so that at least agricultural contribution to the GDP increases as other sectors of economy suffers badly.

Another positive factor related to agricultural produce is food stocking. It should be noted that because of surplus production of crops over the last three years, "massive, excess stock of food grain" has been stocked by the Food Corporation of India (FCI). It is this stock that has been feeding the population during lockdowns.[42] Therefore, it is clear that investment in agricultural production will help India to sustain its economy by employing the recently reverse-migrants to the villages, increase crop production, contribute to GDP, cater to food security and could be used during a crisis situation of the magnitude of the present one facing the world.

To sum up, the government is using various permutations and combinations to come up with a solution to handle this crisis situation. To ease the economy, for instance, the Central Government announced a stimulus package totalling Rs. 20 Lakh Crore that will amount to about 10 per cent of country's GDP. Some experts called the package an all-inclusive pack which gives due importance to all the sectors and barely "leaves any major sphere untouched". Starting from investments in MSMEs and provision of loans to them, for non-bank lenders, employees provident fund, power distribution companies, migrants, street vendors, etc., the list goes on and the package will boost some economy of the country.[43] However, given the population of India, the amount may seem inadequate in the long run. There will be a need for more such stimulus packages especially for the marginalised sections.

While the short-term implications of COVID-19 are multi-directional, its long-term effects will be equally or even more brutal. Nevertheless, as necessity is the mother of invention, this is the time when India should take its sustainable development approach more seriously and should commit itself to achieve it soon.

II. Long-Term Impact

The long-term implications of the pandemic are projections based on the current situation. For instance, as the CMIE viewed that there is a job loss of 27 million youngsters in their 20s and 30s, this aspect has serious long-term repercussions. According to CMIE, "they will have to compete with the new cohorts joining the labour force after them, for fewer jobs".[44] Similarly, there is a serious concern that India may be losing its demographic dividend by not creating new jobs for the new entrants to the job sector. Adding to this, the reverse-migration that has taken place has further moved India 15 years behind.[45]

Similarly, other sectors will suffer in intensity. While the short-term impacts will have an escalation in degree in the long-term, there is also an opportunity for India to reorient its policies and focus more on sustainability aspects as coronavirus is just a prelude to the larger, graver and severe issues that might hit the world eventually. This means that preparedness to tackle such forthcoming situations through pre-emptive measures is the need of the hour. This can be done by investing in sustainable infrastructure, building the resilience for the most vulnerable sections, usage of fiscal mechanisms for recovery and resilience, encourage long-term change in behaviour, and regulate enabling technologies.

While the domestic front can be taken care of by sustainable handling, one more aspect that has re-surfaced and that requires attention is formulation of a well-structured evacuation policy for the country so that fewer losses are incurred on the government exchequer and the country is not caught off guard.

Conclusion

With the current crisis looming over the country, there is indeed a need to redefine the national interests of the country. While India's situation with respect to its economy, society and environment was not very convincing even before the arrival of the pandemic, it has multiplied multi-fold in the present times. India was performing poorly on the hunger and poverty indicators; nevertheless, the lockdowns owing to the pandemic have the tendency to not only increase the number of poor below poverty line, but also adversely affect the employment rate of the country.

With the economy slowing down, unemployment rates increasing and mass reverse-migrations due to loss of job opportunities, India's situation could only be worse if the agricultural sector is not given due attention. While the sector acted as a saving grace because of mass stocking of food grains owing to surplus production in the last three years, further attention to it will help its contribution to the economy, help in employing the migrants who have left for homes and will cater to food security of the country.

Hence, there are short-term and long-term impacts of COVID-19. There is no doubt that the pandemic has made the policy makers realise that there is an immediate need to take the sustainable development approach seriously as it has the capability to answer all the rising problems that the country is facing. However, that will require a huge investment in sustainable infrastructure, time component, usage of advanced technologies, provision of resilience to weaker sections of society and many more. Last, but not the least, the pandemic has also revealed that India is in dire need of a proper evacuation policy and a well-structured one to reduce extra spending on the part of the government.

NOTES

1 UN (United Nations) (2020), "COVID-19 Response," https://www.un.org/en/coronavirus/wellness, accessed online 22 May 2020.

2 Thomas L. Friedman (2020), "Our New Historical Divide: B.C. and A.C. – the World Before Corona and the World After", *The New York Times*, 17 March 2020, https://www.nytimes.com/2020/03/17/opinion/coronavirus-trends.html, accessed online 22 May 2020.

3 Hans Joachim Morgenthau (1952), "Another 'Great Debate': The National Interest of the United States", *The American Political Science Review*, vol. 46, no. 4, pp. 961-988.

4 Ahyousha Khan (2020), "COVID-19 and Future of Non-Traditional Threats to National Security," *Modern Diplomacy*, 30 April 2020, https://moderndiplomacy.eu/2020/04/30/covid-19-and-future-of-non-traditional-threats-to-national-security/, accessed online 21 May 2020.

5 Stephan Blank (2020), "Coronavirus has changed the future of national security forever, Here's How," *EURACTIV*, https://www.euractiv.com/section/defence-and-security/opinion/coronavirus-has-changed-the-future-of-national-security-forever-heres-how/, accessed online 26 May 2020.

6 IMF (2020), "World Economic Outlook, April 2020: The Great Lockdown", *World Economic Report*, https://www.imf.org/en/Publications/WEO/Issues/2020/04/14/weo-april-2020, accessed online 26 May 2020.

7 World Economic Forum (WEF) (2020), "COVID Action Platform," https://www.weforum.org/agenda/2020/04/depression-global-economy-coronavirus/, accessed online 26 May 2020.

8 Here, environment does not necessarily mean only the physical environment but includes, social, economic and political environments as well.

9 H. Brundtland (1987), *Our Common Future*, Oxford: Oxford University Press (for the World Commission on Environment and Development).

10 Manjari Singh (2020), "Sustainable Development" in Kumaraswamy, P. R. (ed.) *The Palgrave Handbook of the Hashemite Kingdom of Jordan*, Singapore: Palgrave Macmillan.

11 UN DESA (2017), "The Sustainable Development Goals Report 2017", https://unstats.un.org/sdgs/report/2017/ accessed online 22 May 2020.

12 World Bank (2018), "Pathways to New Economies and Sustainable Livelihoods," http://documents.worldbank.org/curated/en/524131528837983427/text/TL-SCD-0228B-lowres-03212018.txt, accessed online 26 May 2020.

13 Global Hunger Index (GHI) (2019), "2019 Global Hunger Index by Severity," https://www.globalhungerindex.org/results.html, accessed online 26 May 2020.

14 Navin Anthony (2019), "Poverty Index: India Rank 49", *The Week*, 17 August 2019, https://www.theweek.in/theweek/cover/2019/08/17/poverty-index-india-rank-49.html, accessed online 26 May 2020.

15 NITI Aayog (n.d.), "Sustainable Development Goals," https://niti.gov.in/verticals/sustainable-dev-goals, accessed online 22 May 2020.

16 Bertelsmann Stiftung and Sustainable Development Solutions Network (2019), *Sustainable Development 2019: Transformations to Achieve the Sustainable Development Goals*, Pica Publishing, June, https://s3.amazonaws.com/sustainable development.report/2019/2019_sustainable_development_report.pdf, accessed online 26 May 2020.

17 UN-NITI Aayog (2019), *SDG India: Index and Dashboard 2019-20*, p. 12, https://niti.gov.in/sites/default/files/2019-12/SDG-India-Index-2.0_27-Dec.pdf, accessed online 26 May 2020.

18 Ibid., p. 25.

19 Ibid.

20 Ibid., p. 37.

21 "States Struggling to Control Poverty, Hunger," *The New Indian Express*, 8 January 2020, https://www.newindianexpress.com/nation/2020/jan/08/states-struggling-to-control-poverty-hunger-2086527.html, accessed online 28 May 2020.

22 "India's GDP Growth Rate for 2019-20 Estimated at 5% against 6.8% in FY19," *Business Standard*, 7 January 2020, https://www.business-standard.com/article/economy-policy/gdp-first-advance-estimates-predict-economic-growth-at-5-in-2019-2020-120010700990_1.html, accessed online 27 May 2020.

23 Atari Beiger (2019), "Choking Point: India's Environmental Crisis", *Lowy Institute*, 10 January 2019, https://www.lowyinstitute.org/the-interpreter/choking-point-india-environment-crisis, accessed online 28 May 2020.

24 IMF (2020), "World Economic Outlook," n. 6.

25 Prasanna Mohanty (2020), "Budget 2020: Niti Aayog Shocker; Poverty, Hunger and Income Inequality up in 22 to 25 States and UTs", *Business Today*, 9 January 2020, https://www.businesstoday.in/union-budget-2020/news/budget-2020-niti-

aayog-shocker-poverty-hunger-income-inequality-up-in-22-to-25-states-uts-poor-indians/story/393404.html, accessed online 30 May 2020.

26 World Bank (2020), "COVID-19 Crisis: Through a Migration Lens", Migration and Development Brief 32, April 2020, https://openknowledge.worldbank.org/bitstream/handle/10986/33634/COVID-19-Crisis-Through-a-Migration-Lens.pdf?sequence=5&isAllowed=y, accessed online 28 May 2020.

27 Ibid.

28 "13 Countries, 64 Flights, 3 Navy Warships: How Govt Plans to Bring Back Over 14,000 stranded Indians in Phase I", *The Times of India*, 05 May 2020, https://timesofindia.indiatimes.com/india/13-countries-64-flights-3-navy-warships-how-govt-plans-to-bring-back-over-14000-stranded-indians-in-phase-1/articleshow/75552213.cms, accessed online 29 May 2020.

29 Ministry of External Affairs (2020), "Third Evacuation Flight from Wuhan, China," Government of India, 27 February 2020, https://mea.gov.in/press-releases.htm?dtl/32432/Third+Evacuation+Flight+from+Wuhan+China, accessed online 29 May 2020.

30 "Coronavirus: 263 Indians evacuated from Italy Sent to ITBP Quarantine", *The Economic Times*, 22 March 2020, https://economictimes.indiatimes.com/news/politics-and-nation/coronavirus-263-indians-evacuated-from-italy-sent-to-itbp-quarantine/articleshow/74756441.cms, accessed online 29 May 2020.

31 Manjari Singh (2020), "The Influence of Coronavirus on Diplomatic Relations: Iran, China, Gulf Arabs and India", Fikra Forum, *Washington Institute for Near East Policy (WINEP)*, 21 May 2020, https://www.washingtoninstitute.org/fikraforum/view/Coronavirus-Diplomacy-Trade-Iran-China-Gulf-States-India, accessed online 29 May 2020.

32 Ministry of External Affairs (2020), "Vande Bharat Mission- List of Flights," https://www.mea.gov.in/vande-bharat-mission-list-of-flights.htm, accessed online 30 May 2020.

33 Constantino Xavier (2016), "India's Expatriate Evacuation Operations: Bringing the Diaspora Home", *Carnegie Endowment for International Peace*, December 2016, https://carnegieendowment.org/files/CP_299_Xavier_India_Diaspora_Final.pdf, accessed online 28 May 2020.

34 The World Bank (2020), "COVID-19 Crisis," n. 26.

35 Yogima Seth Sharma (2020), "27 Million Youth In Age Group 20-30 Years Lost Jobs in April: CMIE", *The Economic Times*, 13 May 2020, https://economictimes.indiatimes.com/news/economy/indicators/unemployment-rate-dips-to-23-97-data-from-cmie-shows/articleshow/75689370.cms?from=mdr, accessed online 30 May 2020.

36 Yogima Seth Sharma (2020), "Unemployment Rate in India at 24% for Week Ended May 17: CMIE", *The Economic Times*, 19 May 2020, https://economictimes.indiatimes.com/news/economy/indicators/unemployment-rate-in-india-at-24-for-the-week-ended-may-17-cmie/articleshow/75821968.cms, accessed online 30 May 2020.

37 ILO (2020), "ILO Monitor: COVID-19 and the World of Work", 07 April 2020, https://www.ilo.org/wcmsp5/groups/public/@dgreports/@dcomm/documents/briefingnote/wcms_740877.pdf, accessed online 30 May 2020.

38 "Lockdown in India has Impacted 40 Million Internal Migrants: World Bank", *The*

Economic Times, 23 April 2020, https://economictimes.indiatimes.com/news/politics-and-nation/lockdown-in-india-has-impacted-40-million-internal-migrants-world-bank/articleshow/75311966.cms, accessed online 30 May 2020.

39 Arjun Kumar (2020), "Covid-19 and the Lockdown Impact: Estimating the Unemployment and Job Losses in India's Informal Economy", *The Times of India*, 13 April 2020, https://timesofindia.indiatimes.com/blogs/red-button-day-light/covid-19-and-the-lockdown-impact-estimating-the-unemployment-and-job-losses-in-indias-informal-economy/, accessed online 30 May 2020.

40 Sandhya Keelery (2020), "Estimated Economic Impact from the Coronavirus (Covid-19) on India between April and June 2020, by Sector GVA," *Statista*, 14 May 2020, https://www.statista.com/statistics/1107798/india-estimated-economic-impact-of-coronavirus-by-sector/, accessed online 30 May 2020.

41 Zia Haq (2020), "Farm Sector, Poised to Grow by 3%, Remains a Beacon of Hope Amid Pandemic", *The Hindustan Times*, 24 May 2020, https://www.hindustan times.com/india-news/farm-sector-a-beacon-of-hope-in-economic-gloom/story-YEsFZcYnq76VGI41ic5zz M.html?fbclid=IwAR10qlf E5Sxf8Rb26yqR7OYVJyt OcSGBS4cXN_N4cgY_cYkeKJ_YmGdj-04, accessed online 30 May 2020.

42 Vikas Rawal and Manish Kumar (2020), "COVID-19 Lockdown: The Public Distribution of Food grain", *Coronapolicyimpact.org*, https://coronapolicy impact. org/2020/05/24/covid-19-lockdown-and-the-pds/?fbclid=IwAR16 Hathle StCRdzRgadkN912Wkl1HP4qzwhf9p4Kt-n3WoN6zhbogRO1zw, accessed online 30 May 2020.

43 "Summing Up Modi's Covid Stimulus: Big Takeaways from the Big Covid Package", *The Economic Times*, 17 May 2020, https://economictimes.indiatimes.com/news/economy/policy/summing-up-modis-covid-stimulus-takeaways-so-far-from-the-mother-of-all-incentives/articleshow/75758840.cms?from=mdr, accessed on 30 May 2020.

44 Yogima Seth Sharma (2020), "27 Million Youth In Age Group 20-30 Years Lost Jobs in April: CMIE", *The Economic Times*, 13 May 2020, https://economictimes.india times.com/news/economy/indicators/unemployment-rate-dips-to-23-97-data-from-cmie-shows/articleshow/75689370.cms?from=mdr, accessed online 30 May 2020.

45 Shobana K. Nair (2020), "Reverse Economy to Villages has Set Economy Back by 15 Years, Says JNU Professor", *The Hindu*, 25 May 2020, https://www.the hindu.com/business/Economy/reverse-migration-to-villages-has-set-economy-back-by-15-years-says-jnu-professor/article31671389.ece?utm_source = vuukle&utm_medium=talk_of_town, accessed online 30 May 2020.

3

India's Commerce and Industry: Seeking a Silver Line in the Cloud

RS Sandhu

Hit by COVID-19, the global economy has been devastated following the disruption of the global supply and value chain system. China being the manufacturing hub and the first epicentre of the coronavirus, the resulting lockdown measure to control the virus spread gravely affected the export-import system. Developed countries such as the USA, the United Kingdom, Japan and those of the European Union have been hit drastically, as a large portion of their production activity is based in China and thereby, crippled due to strict lockdown measures. Owing to this domino effect, economists and statisticians have predicted a global economic recession. As per Morgan Stanley, global GDP growth will decelerate by 2.3 per cent over the previous year in the first half of 2020, but would witness a recovery in the second half of the year.[1] Here, it is important to note that the projections of the potential impact of COVID-19 on economies around the globe would not be the same, but vary widely.

In this perspective, in case of India, as UN forecasts suggest, India's projected economic growth is expected to slow to 1.2 per cent in 2020—a further deterioration from the already slowed growth of 4.1 per cent in 2019.[2] While Moody slashed India's GDP growth rate to "zero" for 2020-21 (earlier estimated to be 2.6 per cent); however, it has also forecast that the GDP will bounce back to 6.6 per cent in 2021-22.[3] The other forecasts include Fitch—0.8 per cent; IMF—1.9 per cent; World Bank—1.5-2.8 per cent and ADB—4 per cent.[4] Interestingly, as per the United Nations Conference on Trade and Development (UNCTAD) report, India and China are likely to be exceptions in the predicted global recession.[5]

While on an aggregate basis, trade, hotel, transport, storage and communications sectors are most likely to be affected in FY20/21, international trade will also be affected by several new hurdles due to global lockdowns and restrictions imposed by other countries on exports as well as on imports. Due to which, a fear of contamination through outbound shipments has led to a contraction in exports and imports.

According to India's Commerce Ministry, India's exports rose for the first time in seven months in February growing by 2.91 per cent to US$ 27.65 billion, while the imports also grew by 2.48 per cent to US$ 37.5 billion.[6] All the major foreign exchange earners such as petroleum products, engineering goods and electronic items registered expansion in the month year-on-year. Consequently, the trade deficit fell to US$ 9.85 billion as against US$ 9.72 billion in February 2019. Moreover, the contraction in exports and imports can be seen since March, which coincidentally marks the beginning of the spread of the virus in India.

As observed in the survey conducted by the Federation of Indian Chambers of Commerce and Industry (FICCI), over 50 per cent of Indian companies see the impact on their operations and nearly 80 per cent have witnessed a decline in cash flows.[7] More than 60 per cent affected by the pandemic expect the situation to worsen further, while nearly 42 per cent estimate it to take up to three months for normalcy to return.[8] The restricted import of raw materials from China can delay the normal conditions for businesses in India. The wisdom lies in identifying indigenous suppliers of raw materials as a part of the industrial policy of India and this will likely reduce some quantity and expense and give an internal boost to the slackened trade. In view of which, on 18 May 2020, Indian Prime Minister Narendra Modi put forward the vision of *"Atmanirbhar Bharat Abhiyan"* aimed at creating a self-reliant India.[9] Here, the emphasis is on the need to promote local Indian products and brands to build a robust supply chain that stands the weather of global storms, such as COVID-19.

Here, it is significant to note that despite the tremendous potential, Indian MSMEs are plagued by various other challenges such as poor infrastructure, lack of access to markets and modern technology, inadequate capital and getting statutory clearances related to power, environment, labour, and others. However, the need of the hour lies in boosting the existing systems to enhance the process of India becoming 'self-reliant' in the post-pandemic phase. What also makes self-reliance significant is the fact that the economic losses under COVID-19 has resulted in salary cuts compounded with companies and industries forced to look at major layoffs and downsizing of manpower thus, adding to the social instability.

With India's increasing economic uncertainties and challenges to sustain, the present chapter examines the impact of the pandemic on the Indian economy, especially with focus on the industrial sector. The crux of the paper lies in identifying the opportunities for India to maximise its economic scope in this crisis period and thereafter. In doing so, the chapter will provide a sectoral assessment of India's trade and industry- addressing both the challenges and opportunities under the pandemic.

Impact on India's Industry: *The Highs and Lows of the Lockdown*

India's pharmaceuticals industry has been the biggest beneficiary under COVID-19. The Indian pharmaceutical market (IPM) registered a surprising growth of 8.9 per cent in March 2020 with some evidence of panic buying in chronic medicines.[10] It is important to note that in February, India's domestic pharma market recovered from single-digit growth to a 12.1 per cent growth riding on higher demand for respiratory medicines as well as antibiotics.[11] In addition, eight of the top 10 therapies in the domestic market registered a growth of over 10 per cent.[12]

In the stock market too, shares of pharmaceutical companies are exhibiting promising figures. Such as, among individual stocks, Dr. Reddy's Laboratories, Aurobindo Pharma, Divis Laboratories, Biocon, JB Chemicals & Pharmaceuticals, Caplin Point Laboratories, Aarti Drugs,

Indoco Remedies, RPG Lifesciences and Glenmark Pharmaceuticals were up in the range of 3 per cent to 5 per cent on the National Stock Exchange (NSE).[13] Among key gainers are Cipla that hit a 52-week high of Rs. 651, up 4 per cent in the intra-day trade, while Aurobindo Pharma, too, hit a 52-week high of Rs. 742, up 4 per cent in the intra-day trade.[14]

While the pandemic's obvious 'effect' is witnessed on the pharmaceutical industry, its impact on India's other industries call for a severe crisis- mainly electronic, automobile and travel industries.

I. Electronics Industry: Need for a Reboot

Due to COVID-19, India's electronics industry is battling supply and price issues. With production put to a halt, a wait-and-watch approach is being adopted given the virus outbreak continues. India's electronics industry is highly dependent on China, accounting for 48 per cent of India's manufacturing inputs for electronics, as reported by HDFC.[15] India imported US$ 23.2 billion worth of electrical and electronic items from China in 2018. This is exemplified by the dominance of Chinese smart phones such as Xiaomi, Vivo and Oppo in the Indian market. Thus, the export lockdown has caused an adverse effect on the electronic business.

There is also hope that manufacturing activity will soon pick up and once it resumes, production is likely to be doubled for electronics. But challenges will remain given transport and logistics that will take significant time to come back on track. The automatic impact will be felt in the prices that are likely to shoot up. Given that the lockdown in China will continue to affect the supply chain and quantum of component supplies, it becomes imperative for India to explore alternative supply channels. However, the short supply might cause some negative pressure on prices of these components, resulting in an increase in the prices of products.

For instance, in February 2020, Apple stated the inability to meet its revenue projections due to a decrease in demand and supply, given the lockdown in China As noted, 12 per cent of Apple's handset components are sourced locally in India while 88 per cent are dependent on other overseas countries, with China being a key exporter.[16] Apart from China, India's electronics industry is also dependent on South

Korean companies such as Samsung and the LG Group, which also were severely affected by the coronavirus. South Korea is a substantive base for imported products sold in India.[17]

Hence, India's Electronics Industry needs to find local alternatives or replacements for international products.

II. Brakes on Automobile Industry

COVID-19 led to supply chain disruptions and a production halt in the latter half of March 2020. India's leading automakers such as Mahindra and Mahindra (M&M), Tata Motors and MG Motor India are faced with challenges on component supply from China due to the pandemic. China accounts for 27 per cent of India's automotive part imports.[18] This has resulted in a delay in production and delivery of vehicles like Bharat Stage Four (BS-IV) compliant models.[19] For instance, M&M reported a 42 per cent decline in total sales at 32,476 units in February, added with impact on the Bharat Stage Six (BS-VI) ramp up.[20]

According to Fitch Solutions, vehicle production in India is likely to contract by 8.3 per cent in 2020 following an estimated 13.2 per cent decline in 2019. Thus, India's transition to BS-VI emission norms will be difficult to achieve under the circumstances of the pandemic.[21] This is indicative of a great opportunity for Indian automakers to build and replace imported spare parts using Indian manufacturing bases and such indigenised versions can effectively reduce dependence on foreign goods. This can give a boost to the spare parts industry in India.

III. Travellers' Peril: Effect on the Travel Industry

The impact of coronavirus on the travel and tourism industry is evident through two key factors: cancellation of global events and postponement of vacation plans. Some of the large-format events that stand cancelled as of now include the 2020 Tokyo Olympics, the London Book Fair, the Google News Initiative Global Summit and the Adobe Summit and others affected by both outbound and inbound travel restrictions.

In India, as global companies with offices in India are taking measures to avoid travel, client meetings and off-sites have been turned into video conferences, if not postponed. In lieu of travelling abroad, Indians are now considering domestic vacations. Destinations high in demand include Goa, Himachal Pradesh, Kashmir, Kerala and the Northeast. While neighbouring destinations such as Bhutan, Sri Lanka, Myanmar and Nepal are also gaining popularity. This aspect highlights the increasing tendency among Indian travellers to be cautious with their outbound travel. As online travel aggregator MakeMy Trip (MMT) admitted, a slowdown in outbound travel bookings since the outbreak of coronavirus, such as flight bookings for Southeast Asian countries have been significantly impacted.[22] However, no noticeable dip is yet witnessed in the domestic bookings in India, but it might only be a matter of time before it does.[23] To recover the losses, tourism companies as well as travel and ticket booking agencies are offering flexibility to travellers such as making unlimited changes in travel dates without incurring an extra fee.

Although the recovery will take a considerable time, to cope up with the new uncertainties the travel, tourism and hotel industries need to adapt to the new social distancing norms and introduce contact-free hospitality experiences in the future. The opportunity lies in boosting India's domestic travel to nearby destinations where families can travel in small groups avoiding public gatherings and large crowds at airports and railway stations. The future calls for providing travellers with a safe and COVID-free experience in travel and hospitality.

Plan Ahead for Post-COVID-19: *Acclimatise the New Normal*

I. FMCG: To Stay Relevant, Act Innovative

Across India, in the wake of the pandemic and the lockdown measures, businesses, big and small, are seriously rethinking how to transform themselves to survive this crisis. While companies such as Hindustan Unilever Limited (HUL), PVR and Pidilite are looking at conserving cash to save themselves, retailers such as Arvind, Croma and Titan are setting up a robust omni-channel business model while mall owners such as DLF and Nexus are preparing to go all out to reassure consumers that shopping with them is viable and safe.[24] Given the uncertainty attached and no predictability of the fate of business, risk management has become high on agenda. With the tendency to mostly work on three to five-year plans and yearly budgets, the pandemic calls for a shift towards thinking short-term over long-term planning.

Amidst the pandemic, the biggest challenge faced by companies is mainly two-fold: 'how to sustain themselves' and 'how to stay relevant'. With earnings almost zero, and the new norms of social distancing with people largely staying indoors, businesses are looking for innovative means to stay afloat. Thus, to stay relevant, businesses need to let loose their imagination. This has forced companies to look at strategic tweaks to their existing business model that includes considering ways to re-imagine and re-invent ways of doing business in the pre and post-pandemic periods.

Companies are opting for diversification by going beyond their scope of production. One of the visible trends is noticed in the manufacturing of health and hygiene products. For instance, companies such as HUL, Marico, Godrej and others have diversified their production into manufacturing disinfectants, surface cleaners, sanitizers, germ-free technology based appliances and others, offering a variety of hygiene and safety related options to consumers. To add, foam manufacturers are using Neem Freshe Technology and air mesh fabric in the mattresses to repel allergens and prevent the breeding of microbes. The other visible trend of diversification is noticed in the food business. For instance, India's top luxury hotel chains such as Oberoi, Hyatt, Taj and others have started takeaway and home delivery options to create an alternate source of revenue amidst the crisis.[25] Restaurants are working on virtual menus and have spread out seating. With eating at home becoming the norm, food companies such as GITS, Licious, iD Fresh and Tasty Treat are trying out more ready-to-cook options.[26]

Apart from diversification, companies are also adopting new means in terms of distribution. The bigger challenge for FMCG majors to re-imagine the supply chain and distribution network, given the total stop under lockdown. Here, the question is that of 'survival'. To cope up, FMCG players have tied up with various third-party service providers such as food delivery platforms such as Swiggy, Zomato and Dunzo; cab aggregators and facility management providers of residential complexes to ensure their products reach consumers. This swift change has called for the need to reinvent and make the existing supply chain and distribution networks less prone to shocks such as COVID-19.

Despite the changes, some sectors are facing grave challenges; neither diversification nor distribution can help recover the losses. For instance, the retail sector,[27] which accounts for 40 per cent of consumption, took a US$ 30 billion hit due to COVID-19 in March and has been out of business for all of April and much of May.[28] Liquidity in the retail businesses is driven by seasonal sales and collections, and with the fixed expenditures being stagnant, yet high, the seasonal inflow of cash is what keeps these companies afloat. Absence of this inflow threatens the existence of businesses at large.

With these conditions, survivability has become a bigger concern for the retail giants. For instance, a lifestyle major like The Titan Company is posed with the challenge of how to attract a person sitting at home to buy a piece of jewellery, watch or perfume. With all its retail stores forced to shut down, the company is using the virtual route to appeal to consumers. Under COVID-19, with contamination being a major cause of concern in the mind of the consumer, demand for showroom goods is declining magnanimously - calling for the need to switch to the online sector.

With the world going in for 'contact-less' options, consumers are likely to spend more time online for the purchase of the choicest brands in their quest to avoid the routine visit to the local store. In the light of this, online sales are predicted to surge as and when restrictions are lifted as the rational consumer is on the watch for safer alternatives to shopping. Given 'going contactless' is becoming the new norm, it makes it imperative to digitally empower the *'kiranas'*, local grocery stores, to recover from the economic setback. To aid this process, Shikhar app has been created to enable a grocer to place orders; while an app called "Humara Shop" is in process to help *kiranas* go digital.[29] This further proves that in the post-COVID world, digital solutions in distribution and manufacturing will not only become necessary' but also take precedence.

What calls for such changes? It is not just convenience, but maintaining strong hygiene standards-, which is the most important criterion to be fulfilled by the industry sector, in all areas. Besides, with new trends at play, for the companies to remain relevant, it has become important to understand consumer behaviour, mainly in terms of their consumption and most importantly, their relative relevance in the post-COVID world. Hence, with these innovative measures in action, one can suggest that India has already taken its first step forward in acclimatising under the new norm of living with a pandemic.

II. Make in India: MSMEs as Game Changers

It is well-noted that in the post-lockdown phase with travel bans lifted, there is likely to be a rapid increase in the demand for products from numerous affected nations, especially those dependent on the global supply chain. Here, India should take the opportunity to access the markets in these countries and fill the gap by exporting MSME products to them. This will help overcome the long-standing lack of India's access to markets. The present crisis offers India an opportunity as mentioned earlier in various sectors, especially the MSME, to provide a boost to the 'Make in India' programme and realise the vision of *"Atmanirbhar Bharat Abhiyan"*.

Figure 3.1: Key Industry Shares for MSME (in percentage)

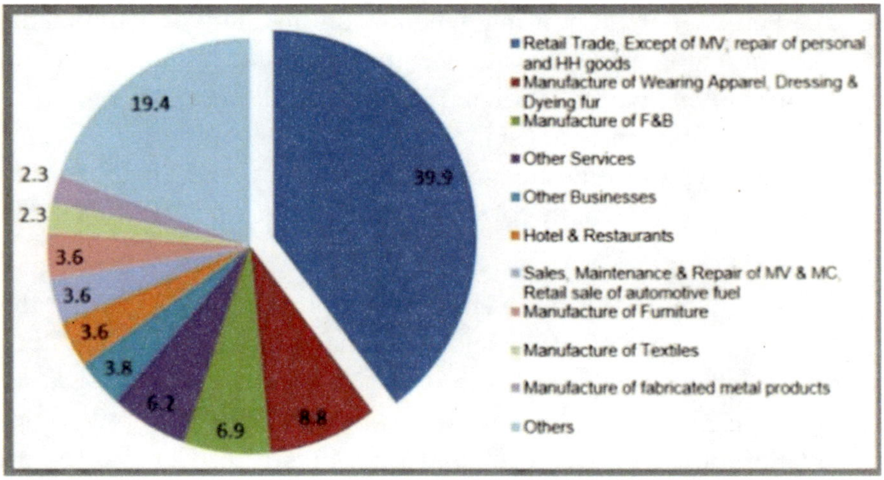

Source: Adapted from Resurgent India.[30]

In accordance with the *Atmanirbhar Bharat Abhiyan*, the five pillars that will serve as foundations for a self-reliant India are:[31] (a) Economy-need for a self-sustaining and indigenous economy, (b) Infrastructure-need in infrastructure to boost supply chain and consolidate it locally, (c) System-need for a system which is simple and quick to respond to all business needs without red-tape, (d) Democracy-the need to guard against panic and fake news in these difficult times and support the concept of a democratic welfare state for all, and (e) Demand-need to generate liquidity in the market in order to boost demand and support for local industry along with increasing per capita purchasing power and providing sustainable employment.

In view of this, to make India's defence sector self-reliant, the Indian government has charted a set of practical measures to boost indigenisation in defence. The major steps taken are:[32] First, increase in FDI via auto route from 49 to 74 per cent without approval from MoD/RBI, which means more investment in on-going and upcoming projects. Second, incorporation of ordnance factory boards (OFBs) to make them autonomous and improving functionality and quality of work and later listing them on the stock exchange. Third, setting up committees for contract management for faster progress of contracts. Fourth, listing the platforms for exclusive Indian production and no joint ventures. Fifth, listing the spares of foreign platforms for indigenous production to save Forex. Sixth, honouring general staff qualitative requirements (GSQRs) of ongoing projects and encouraging Make in India. Seventh, increasing private participation in ISRO. Eight, allowing use of DRDO labs to private players to assist in timely testing of equipment. Ninth, a separate budget for Domestic Capital Procurement. And finally, a list of equipment banned from import to be circulated to encourage Make in India.[33]

What is noteworthy is the emerging importance of MSMEs in the post-lockdown phase that will not only make India 'self-reliant', but also provide a significant boost to India's home-grown industrial and economic sectors. In this process, the Ministry of MSME should work in collaboration with the MEA and the Ministry of Commerce and Industry (MCI) to increase the contribution of India's MSMEs to global trade. To do so, the MEA should identify international demand for specific products in these critical times and the MCI should implement export promotion measures for MSMEs and Ministry of MSME should recognise the potential domestic suppliers, such as those MSMEs involved in the production of essential goods and services and are in high demand. Furthermore, a platform should be created which would give them relevant information regarding access to new markets, and enable them to compete globally. Hence, these steps will improve autonomy, accountability and efficiency in India's defence sector.

India's Post-Lockdown Action Plan: *A Silver Lining in the Policy Reforms*

Given the unfolding reforms because of the COVID-19 pandemic, India's policies in various industries and sectors are likely to witness the following changes:

- *Fast-track Investment Clearances*: Through Empowered Group of Secretaries.
- *Upgradation of Industrial Infrastructure*: Schemes will be implemented in states through challenge mode for industrial cluster upgradation of common infrastructure facilities, communication and connectivity.
- *Government focus on eight sectors*: Coal, Minerals, Defence Production, Airspace Management, Social Infrastructure Projects, Power Distribution Companies, Space Sectors and Atomic Energy.
- *Coal Sector*: Government is introducing commercial mining of coal. India needs to reduce import of substitutable coal and increase self-reliance in production. Nearly 50 blocks will be auctioned. The investment of Rs. 50,000 crore is for the evacuation of enhanced CIL's (Coal India Limited) target of 1 billion tons of coal production by 2023-24 plus coal production from private blocks.
- *Minerals*: Enhancing private investment in mineral sector. Finance Minister Nirmala Sitharaman also explained the rationalisation of stamp duty payable at the time of award of mining leases. 500 mining blocks would be offered through an open and transparent auction process. Joint auction of bauxite and coal mineral blocks will be introduced to enhance the aluminium industry's competitiveness.

- *Defence Production*: Enhancing self-reliance in defence production, Indigenization of imported spares, separate budget provisioning for domestic capital procurement. These steps will improve autonomy, accountability and efficiency in the sector. Foreign Direct Investment limit in defence manufacturing under automatic route is being raised from 49 per cent to 74 per cent. Corporatisation of Ordnance Factory Board was also proposed.
- *Civil Aviation (Airspace Management, World Class Airports Through PPP, MRO Hub)*: Restrictions on the utilisation of Indian air space will be eased so that civilian flying becomes more efficient. The effort will bring a total benefit of Rs. 1,000 crore per year for the aviation sector. Construction of world-class airports through PPP route. Government is working hard to make India a global hub for aircraft maintenance, repair and overhaul. The Airports Authority of India has awarded three airports out of six bids for operation and maintenance on (PPP) basis. Additional investment by private players in 12 airports in first and second rounds expected around Rs. 13,000 crore.
- *Power Sector Reforms*: Power distribution companies in Union Territories to be privatised in line with the new tariff policies. This will enable us to strengthen industries and bring in efficiency in the entire power sector. This will also enable stability in the sector.
- *Boosting Private Sector Investment*: Boosting private sector investment in Social Infrastructure through revamped and new Viability Gap Funding Scheme of Rs. 8,100 crore.
- *Space Sector*: Boosting private participation in space sector. Government is working on a liberal geo-spatial policy. Private sector to be co-traveller in India's space sector journey through launches, satellite services.
- *Atomic Energy*: The government intends to link India's robust start-up ecosystem to the nuclear sector, Technology Development and Incubation centres will be set up for fostering synergy between research facilities and tech entrepreneurs. Establishment of research reactor in PPP mode for production of medical isotopes.

Conclusion

The Indian Government's efforts to deal with the COVID-19 crisis by promptly enforcing a lockdown, keeping in mind that even developed nations have been unable to cope with this crisis as effectively, is highly appreciated. However, what also needs attention is that the functioning of Indian businesses and industries should not be ignored for much longer. This makes policies, exemptions, and support packages from the Indian government an urgent 'need of the hour'. In this process, management and co-ordination would be the key for policymakers to turn the tables in favour of India by increasing its share in world trade, and steering the growth of the Indian economy.

As the entire economy is standing at the edge of an exponential downfall; it is either going to be a full-blown crash or a moderately safe crash landing, hopefully the latter. In this situation, it is imperative for India to act promptly and take practical measures in order to sustain both its economy and its people.

NOTES

1 Chitranjan Kumar (2020), "Coronavirus impact: Morgan Stanley expects deep global recession, cuts growth by 2.3% for H1FY20", *Business Today*, 30 March 2020, https://www.businesstoday.in/current/economy-politics/coronavirus-impact-morgan-stanley-expects-deep-global-recession-cuts-growth-by-23-for-h1fy20/story/399632.html, accessed online 15 May 2020.

2 "India's growth rate projected to slow to 1.2% in 2020: UN report", *Financial Express*, 13 May 2020, https://www.financialexpress.com/economy/coronavirus-covid19-pandemic-indias-growth-rate-projected-to-slow-to-1-2-in-2020-un-report/1958261/, accessed online 20 May 2020.

3 "Moody slashes India's GDP growth to 'zero' in FY21", *Business Line*, 08 May 2020, https://www.thehindubusinessline.com/economy/moodys-investors-service-sees-indias-economic-growth-at-zero-in-fy21/article31532688.ece, accessed online 15 May 2020.

4 Ibid.

5 "World economy will go into recession with likely exception of India, China: United Nations", *The Economic Times*, 02 April 2020, https://economictimes.indiatimes.com/news/economy/indicators/world-economy-will-go-into-recession-with-likely-exception-of-india-china-united-nations/articleshow/74905696.cms?from=mdr, accessed online 20 May 2020.

6 "Exports post first rise in 7 months, grow by 2.91% in February", *The Economic Times*, 13 March 2020, https://economictimes.indiatimes.com/news/economy/foreign-trade/exports-post-first-rise-in-7-months-grow-by-2-91-in-february/articleshow/74614921.cms?from=mdr, accessed online 15 May 2020.

7 "Coronavirus impact: Over 50% of India Inc sees impact on ops, 80% witness fall in cash flow", *The Economic Times*, 20 March 2020, https://economictimes.indiatimes.com/news/economy/indicators/coronavirus-impact-over-50-of-india-inc-sees-impact-on-ops-80-witness-fall-in-cash-flow/articleshow/74726229.cms?from=mdr, accessed online 15 May 2020.

8 Ibid.

9 "Atmanirbhar Bharat Abhiyan: PM Modi urges nation to buy and promote local", *The Economic Times*, 12 May 2020, https://economictimes.indiatimes.com/news/politics-and-nation/atmanirbhar-bharat-abhiyan-pm-modi-urges-nation-to-buy-and-promote-local/videoshow/75701635.cms?from=mdr, accessed online 16 May 2020.

10 Cardiac registered a monthly growth of 19.8 per cent compared to 11.0 per cent in February 2020, Anti-Diabetic registered growth of 18.2 per cent compared to 11.0 per cent in February 2020 and Respiratory medicines grew at a 22.9 per cent compared to 11.5 per cent in February 2020. See, Sohini Das (2020), "Coronavirus outbreak: Pharma market grows 9% in March due to panic buying", *Business Standard*, 09 April 2020, https://www.business-standard.com/article/companies/panic-buying-amid-coronavirus-lockdown-helped-pharma-market-grow-9-120040801570_1.html, accessed online 16 May 2020.

11 Ibid.

12 Ibid.

13 "Pharma shares in focus: Cipla, Aurobindo Pharma hit 52-week high", *Business Standard*, 29 May 2020, https://www.business-standard.com/article/markets/pharma-shares-in-focus-cipla-aurobindo-hit-52-week-highs-120052900607_1.html, accessed online 31 May 2020.

14 Ibid.

15 Pranit Sarda and Naini Thaker (2020), "Electronics sector battles supply and price issues as production halts in China", *Forbes India*, 06 March 2020, https://www.forbesindia.com/article/leaderboard/electronics-sector-battles-supply-and-price-issues-as-production-halts-in-china/58143/1, accessed online 15 May 2020.

16 Ibid.

17 Ibid.

18 "Coronavirus' impact on India's auto sector," *The Economic Times*, 10 April 2020, https://economictimes.indiatimes.com/markets/stocks/news/coronavirus-whats-its-impact-on-indias-auto-sector/articleshow/75078607.cms?from=mdr, accessed online 15 May 2020.

19 Ibid.

20 Tata Motors, M&M, MG Motors face supply issues from China over coronavirus", *Business Standard*, 01 March 2020, https://www.business-standard.com/article/pti-stories/tata-motors-m-m-mg-motor-say-coronavirus-outbreak-in-china-impacting-parts-supply-120030100672_1.html, accessed online 14 May 2020.

21 Ibid.

22 "Witnessing slowdown in outbound travel bookings amid coronavirus: MakeMyTrip", *The Economic Times*, 04 March 2020, https://economictimes.indiatimes.com/industry/services/travel/witnessing-slowdown-in-outbound-travel-bookings-amid-coronavirus-makemytrip/articleshow/74480742.cms?from=mdr, accessed online 17 May 2020.

23 Ibid.

24 Ajitha Shashidhar and Sonal Khetarpal (2020), "Transform or Die", *Business Today*, 31 May 2020, https://www.businesstoday.in/magazine/cover-story/transform-or-die/story/403598.html, accessed online 31 May 2020.

25 See, Nisha Shroff (2020), "Indian luxury hotels tap into food delivery segment," *Business Traveller*, 08 April 2020, https://www.businesstraveller.com/business-travel/2020/04/08/indian-luxury-hotels-tap-into-food-delivery-segment/, accessed online 20 May 2020.

26 Sonal Khetarpal (2020), "Demand for ready-to-eat meals spikes amid coronavirus lockdown", *Business Today*, 07 May 2020, https://www.businesstoday.in/latest/trends/demand-for-ready-to-eat-meals-spikes-amid-coronavirus-lockdown/story/403180.html, accessed online 16 May 2020.

27 Given the circumstances, it is estimated that the industry will take at least six months to get back on track in terms of cash inflows; but only if companies can actually survive this downfall in the next six months. Additionally, the losses over six months can cross a figure of about $ 700 billion (estimated from the $ 30 billion fortnight) and the recovery period of these losses can be well over a decade for some businesses.

28 Abhinav Singh (2020), "Retailers lost $ 30 billion from lockdown, labour shortage likely in future: Experts", *The Week*, 03 April 2020, https://www.theweek.in/news/biz-tech/2020/04/03/retailers-lost-30-billion-from-lockdown-labour-shortage-likely-in-future-experts1.html, accessed online 16 May 2020.

29 Ajitha Shashidhar and Sonal Khetarpal (2020), "Transform or Die", n. 24.

30 See, "MSME Sector in India - The Engine of Growth (Contribution of MSME in the GDP) - Part-3," *Resurgent India*, 24 April 2015, https://www.slideshare.net/ResurgentIndia/msme-sector-in-india-the-engine-of-growth-part-3, accessed online 31 May 2020.

31 "PM Modi shares five pillars that will make India self-reliant in Covid-19 times," *India Today*, 12 May 2020, https://www.indiatoday.in/india/story/pm-modi-speech-5-pillars-atm-nirbhar-india-self-reliance-covid-19-lockdown-1677293-2020-05-12, accessed online 16 May 2020.

32 Manu Pubby (2020), "Separate budget for Indian made defence items, negative import list: FM Nirmala Sitharaman", *The Economic Times*, 16 May 2020, https://economictimes.indiatimes.com/news/defence/fm-announces-hike-in-fdi-in-defence-production-ban-on-certain-imports-of-defence-weapons/articleshow/75775687.cms?from=mdr, accessed online 18 May 2020.

33 Ibid.

4

India at the Global High Table: With Great Power Comes Great Responsibility

Amrita Jash

The COVID-19 pandemic has brought to the surface the ground rule of international politics that there are 'no permanent friends, or permanent enemies, but only permanent interests'. This has added to the competitive dynamics between the great powers that has led to 'tote-board' or 'scorecard' diplomacy in times of crisis. In this case, both the interests and scores are driven by which country is effective in tackling the health crisis. In addition, with the WHO under severe scrutiny for its leadership over the handling of the pandemic, a coordinated approach at the international level, has been superseded by an individual national approach with countries tackling the crisis in their own way. The caveat lies in the fact that with each country maintaining social distancing, imposing countrywide lockdowns, and holding commercial restrictions on travel and trade has only provided a temporary fix to the pandemic; but has failed to offer a long-term solution to the global tragedy of the commons.

Causing turmoil, the circumstances of the rapid spread of the virus has raised significant alarms over the stability of the existing world order. That is, on one end, the overwhelmed health care system compounded with increased distress to the global economy has brought the functioning of the international system to a standstill; on the other end, with China under scrutiny over the Wuhan epidemic, has surfaced the growing global divide over handling of the pandemic. This is highlighted in the growing global criticism of China over its lack of transparency and reluctance to act during the early stages of the virus outbreak.

One of the crucial aspect that is adding to the COVID-19 disaster is the Sino-US rift, which has resulted into a competitive dynamic between the two great powers. The turf battle, as highlighted in US President Donald Trump's calling the virus as "Chinese virus" added with allegations of "mask diplomacy" and "faulty" Chinese test kits, has been rebutted with Beijing's counter charge on the "US army of bringing the epidemic to Wuhan". The war of the narratives has resulted into a united front based on 'blame China' and 'make China pay'—thus, impacting every nation that is party to the international order. Apart from the WHO, the United Nations Security Council's (UNSC) delayed and inconclusive approach towards the pandemic has further highlighted the insufficiency- adding to the growing speculations over the efficiency and relevance of such international institutions in handling global crises.

The implications of which have prompted shifts in the international order, as most countries are re-thinking their ties with Beijing as well as re-evaluating the role of international institutions. By posing a severe challenge to the existing international order, COVID-19 pandemic has resulted into a global disorder. Wherein, the strategic shifts are calling for: the emergence of a new world order, namely, the 'post-pandemic world order'; changes in the global balance of power catalysed by the de-coupling of Sino-American ties; re-defining of traditional understanding of national security; extension of the envelope of national interest and, above all, re-evaluating national security preparedness. Thereby, countries must prepare themselves as the world is entering into an uncharted territory.

Against this backdrop, it becomes imperative to understand the changing dynamics of India's role in the global order. More importantly, after succeeding Japan, in May 2020 India took over as the next Chairperson of the 34-member WHO Executive Board,[1] wherein the challenge for India at the high table lies in proving to be 'responsible'.

Here, the timing of India's appointment is crucial, against the worldwide debate and criticism on the role played by WHO as the world's pandemic watchdog compounded with allegations against WHO Director-General Tedros Adhanom Ghebreyesus of playing into China's hands over the coronavirus. What adds to India's pressure is the growing calls for a global enquiry, especially from the USA and Australia to investigate the source of origin of the virus in Wuhan and Beijing's subsequent action on it.

In view of this, under the prevailing uncertainty and severity of the global situation, the bigger query remains: What are the new contours that define a responsible global actor? For, in the post-COVID world order, if a nation claims to call itself responsible, then the stakes are higher than ever. In this context of contested responsibility, the present chapter aims to assess the impact of COVID-19 on India's role in the global order. The key pointers of examination are India's actions under COVID-19 and how it is likely to shape India's role as a global actor in the post-COVID world order.

India Re-defines its Global Role: *Pragmatic, Proactive and Responsible*

When the world's major players such as USA and Europe proved to be a failure in handling the virus outbreak as witnessed in their crumbled healthcare system and unprecedented rate of fatality, India proved to be an exception in many ways. Despite its 1.3 billion population and holding the status of a 'developing country', India proved to incur comparatively less damage both in terms of number of infections and most importantly lower fatality rate by withstanding the world's largest nationwide lockdown. The other aspect that makes India an exception amidst the pandemic is New Delhi's emergence as an engaged and active global player in fighting the health crisis. Instead, rather than adopting an individualist approach, India under the leadership of Prime Minister Narendra Modi promoted the collective approach in fighting the pandemic.

I. Setting a Global Tone to the Handling of the Pandemic

On 11 March, WHO declared COVID-19 a global "pandemic,"[2] to which, India acted proactively by calling for a joint fight in the South Asian region. On 13 March, Prime Minister Modi pitched the proposal in a social media message by tweeting, "I would like to propose that the leadership of SAARC [South Asian Association for Regional Cooperation] nations chalk out a strong strategy to fight Coronavirus".[3] Most notably, in outlaying a significant but surprise diplomatic move, Modi proposed a "video conference" among leaders of Afghanistan, Pakistan, Bangladesh, Nepal, Bhutan, Maldives and Sri Lanka to discuss a strategy to combat the disease in the region.[4] With this diplomatic move, India aimed to "set an example to the world" as emphasised in the tweet, of a united fight against the virus. India's intention of acting with responsibility did succeed in setting a global precedent as proposal received an immediate positive response from all South Asian states, including Pakistan despite its political differences with India. Acting on India's call, a video conference of the leaders of SAARC was convened on 15 March[5]—underscoring the need for "regional coordination to address complex cross-border challenges".[6]

Emphasising the need for coordinated efforts to adequately address the global challenge, India put forward a five-point proposal to help other South Asian nations, suggesting:[7] First, establishing a SAARC Emergency Response Fund for COVID-19, with an initial US$ 10 million contribution from India. Second, follow-up discussions between medical professionals of the SAARC region, as well as trade and economic officials, to assess the impact of the pandemic. Third, deploying India's specially-constituted Rapid Response Teams of medical and other professionals, and testing equipment, to any SAARC nation with additional support for capacity-building.[8] Fourth, sharing India's software for integrated health information for disease surveillance. Fifth, and lastly, offering support by the Indian Council for Medical Research (ICMR) for a platform of the SAARC States to share ideas for diagnostic and the therapeutic intervention for epidemics.[9]

India's regional approach acted as a booster in reflecting and elevating India's responsible attitude as a global actor. To argue so, first, India's SAARC vision provided an impetus to regional institutions, which is criticised of being irrelevant and defunct in South Asia's regional dynamics. However, with all seven South Asian nations acting in unison to India's call did provide a thrust to revamp the role of SAARC as well as reinstated India's role as a regional leader. And second, Modi's vision provided a boost to India's global role as no other world leader, neither the USA, China or the European Union, adopted either a regional or a global outlook towards the pandemic; rather these countries represented a home-bound approach, while India's exceptional outlook positioned it both as a leader and architect of a global response to COVID-19 along with combating it at home. The virtual SAARC meeting is both symbolic and significant in reflecting India's proactive diplomacy in times of global crisis—as it set a new precedent of virtual diplomacy in the international system.

Further extending the scope of India's diplomatic outreach from the regional level, India made the second stint at the global level. On 17 March, Prime Minister Modi, in a telephonic conversation with Saudi Crown Prince Mohammed bin Salman (the current G20 Chair) proposed the possibility of replicating the SAARC web conference format to the G20 forum.[10] India's proposal culminated in the "Extraordinary Virtual G20 Leaders' Summit" convened on 26 March to discuss the challenges of the pandemic and forge a global coordinated response.[11] Emphasising on the need for a global response to fight the pandemic, the "G20 Leaders' Statement" categorically stated: "The unprecedented COVID-19 pandemic is a powerful reminder of our interconnectedness and vulnerabilities. The virus respects no borders. [In] Combating this pandemic [...] We are strongly committed to presenting a united front against this common threat"—calling for measures to safeguard the global economy, minimising trade disruption and steps to enhance global cooperation.[12]

Taking a step forward, India at the Virtual Summit, called for the promotion of new crisis management protocols and procedures for an interconnected global village and emphasised on the importance to strengthen and reform intergovernmental organisations like the WHO.[13] India's vision has been validated by the series of virtual G20 ministerial events as held in April-May 2020 that spanned from tracks on energy, agriculture, digital economy, labour and employment tourism, and trade and investment.[14]

What made India's responsive approach towards proposing a G20 virtual summit imperative is the fact that G20 comprises of 85 per cent of the global economy. As per OECD, all G20 economies in 2020 will face a downward revision given the adverse impact on confidence, financial markets, the travel sector and disruption to supply chains.[15] This timely approach in taking stock of the risks provided clarity, as is deemed necessary to alleviate the unwarranted economic disruptions. For instance, in a pre-emptive response, the G20 nations injected over US$ 5 trillion into the global economy as part of targeted fiscal policy, economic measures, and guarantee schemes to counteract the social, economic and financial impacts of the pandemic.[16] Adding to G20's measures, the International Monetary Fund and the Word Bank jointly called for suspension of debt payments from developing countries to avert risks of debt vulnerabilities due by the pandemic.[17]

With these overtures, it can be argued that India's proactive leadership helped shape and adopt a global vision towards the handling of the pandemic. To which, speculations have been raised suggesting that India's global appeal on a coordinated response is likely to lose its traction given most countries are focused on dealing with the coronavirus at home.[18] What can add to it is India's own worsening situation at home that could prompt New Delhi to abandon its global outreach and become homebound, just as others. However, against these speculations, it can also be argued that India's responsive call for a global action did come as a timely measure—highlighting the need to re-boot the old global systems to fight the 'new age' pandemic, as no country can champion winning over the virus on its own.

II. Extending a Helping Hand by Dialling Up Medical Diplomacy

In addition to championing ideas of virtual meetings of global leaders, India's fight against COVID-19 is also represented by its medical assistance to various countries to combat the pandemic. For instance, countries in India's immediate neighbourhood such as Maldives, Sri Lanka, Mauritius and Seychelles were among the first nations to receive India's medical aid, added with considering aid requests from Italy and Iran—two of the world's hardest-hit countries. While Maldives, Mauritius, Comoros and Kuwait have also received medical rapid response teams from India to augment the preparedness in tackling the pandemic. Also, India had evacuated nine Maldives nationals from

China's Wuhan—which was once the epicentre of the coronavirus outbreak.

In due time, India's Ministry of External Affairs had already pledged to supply drugs, testing kits and other medical assistance worth Rs. 60 crore to 67 countries—in addition to the drugs and equipment that India supplies to various countries on commercial terms.[19] Of the 67 countries, India has sent consignments worth Rs. 28 crore to 29 countries across the South Asian region, the Indian Ocean region, the Gulf (Kuwait), Central Asia (Kazakhstan, Armenia, Tajikistan and Ukraine) and remotely-located countries like the Dominican Republic and Ecuador as well as six more African countries.[20] However, with increasing requests of assistance from countries, India broadened the cover to over 90-plus countries with an estimated cost of Rs. 110-120 crore (Rs. 1.1-1.2 billion).[21]

What is noteworthy is that to help aid the fight against COVID-19, India lifted its export ban on drugs such as hydroxychloroquine (HCQ) (seen by some as a possible cure for COVID-19) and paracetamol in a bid to supply them to other countries. For instance, in April, India supplied 85 million HCQ tablets and close to 500 million paracetamol tablets to 108 countries,[22] of which, 5 million HCQ tablets and a large quantity of paracetamol has been allotted to 31 countries as grant assistance to combat COVID-19.[23] Specifically, 80 million HCQ tablets were supplied to 24 countries through commercial contracts including the USA, UK, Russia, France, Spain and The Netherlands; large quantities of paracetamol tablets were supplied to 52 countries including Italy, Sweden and Singapore; and in some cases, both tablets were supplied.[24]

What is noteworthy is that despite the travel bans in place, India has managed to carry forward its diplomatic outreach of medical assistance across the globe. The consignments have been dispatched by special Indian Air Force flights, foreign evacuation charters and as diplomatic cargo. For instance, India dispatched HCQ tablets to the Dominican Republic via diplomatic cargo on a US evacuation flight to Atlanta, Georgia; to Mauritius and Seychelles on special Indian Air Force planes and to Afghanistan by a special charter.[25]

Notably, India's Armed Forces have been actively engaged in carrying forward India's mission abroad. For instance, in February, Indian Air Force (C17) relief aircraft evacuated 76 Indians and 36 foreign nationals[26] from Wuhan—the then epicentre of the coronavirus.[27] Furthermore, the Indian Air Force in cooperation with the Indian Army launched an 18-hour "Operation Sanjeevani" to deliver 6.2 tonnes of essential medicines and hospital consumables to the Maldives.[28] While the Indian Navy has been involved in carrying New Delhi's diplomatic outreach to the Indian Ocean countries. India's warship INS Khatri (5,600-tonne landing ship) deployed under "Mission Sagar" has carried medical teams, consignments of essential medicines and food supplies to Maldives, Mauritius, Madagascar, Comoros and Seychelles.[29]

With these overtures, New Delhi's fast track approach in extending help despite the challenge at home has elevated India's role both symbolically as well as significantly. The COVID-19 crisis has further proved India's mettle as the first responder to any crisis not just in the region but also globally. Highlighting India's dedicated approach, New Delhi's initiatives to render assistance has exemplified its readiness to combat an emergency situation both through manpower and resources. Most importantly, it has validated India's responsive approach to its immediate and extended neighbourhood.

India in the Post-COVID World Order: *A Confident, Strong and Responsible Stakeholder*

In the backdrop of the systemic turmoil, COVID-19 has highlighted the crisis of leadership in the international order as major powers are practising 'each to their own' policy. This has put the international system in a state of flux. Taking lessons from the chaos, it becomes imperative in the post-COVID world to set the priorities right. The right mix entails that healthcare, education, environment, and terms of trade must be given priority as equated with nuclear disarmament, the global financial system, and multi-polarity; added with undertaking of significant reforms of global institutions such as the UN and other bodies.

India's middle-power status has often left it ignored or not being taken seriously at the global high table. However, with new-found interest to assert its importance and place in the world under the pandemic, India's role and status are experiencing a significant shift. For India's low key attitude has often raised speculations over being acknowledged as a 'rising power'. But, the pandemic has called for a shift—both in India's attitude as well as in that of others towards India. Stepping up as a leader in shaping a global fight towards COVID-19 when the world's leading powers acted otherwise, India has ably demonstrated its preparedness, capability and wisdom in handling the pandemic—thus, dispelling the speculations over its calibre to be a global actor. In contrast to China's image as a global player that is under review over its handling of the Wuhan epidemic, India has experienced a boost to its global image by championing the call for a global fight against the pandemic as a responsible player. Also, India's modest actions have earned it the recognition of being credible. In the new world, India's role is likely to witness an expansion beyond the usual—no more just participatory, but taking the lead in many ways.

In view of this, the post-COVID world order is likely to witness a greater manoeuvring space for India. With uncertainty over how the post-COVID world would look like, what is certain is that a 'new world' is in the making, to which old principles do not apply. With greater multi-polarity, it is multilateralism that will gain more traction, as power will no more be limited only to a privileged few. In view of this, some of India's top table decision-making is likely to be witnessed in the following quarters.

I. India at the WHO

Given its premier appointment at a crucial timing, the big question for New Delhi is: What will India do at the WHO? But, what can be called a twist to the tale is the question—'What can India do at the WHO?' India's decision-making will be tested on two key fronts: first, the looming global pressure to seek an investigation on the spread of the virus since its inception in Wuhan. Second, the Taiwan aspect in support of the US move to reinstate Taiwan's observer status at the World Health Assembly (WHA).

India has already acted on its first choice. On 18 May, at the WHA meeting, India along with 61 other nations moved the proposal[30] to "identify the zoonotic source" asking for an "impartial, independent and comprehensive evaluation" of the WHO's response to COVID-19.[31] It is widely acknowledged that the virus originated in China's Wuhan given that the first COVID-19 case was reported in Wuhan in December 2019. However, Beijing has refuted this theory, as on 12 May, the Chinese Embassy in India's spokesperson, Ji Rong, tweeted: "#Wuhan city in #China first reported COVID19 cases, but that does not mean the virus originated in Wuhan. [..] It is irresponsible to connect the virus with Wuhan and stigmatize China".[32] Against its opposition to an arbitrary investigation based on "presumption of guilt,"[33] China has recently indicated support for a review but "at an appropriate time after the pandemic is over".[34] Here, the contestation lies on the terms and conditions of the enquiry of the virus. With this choice, India took its first decision at the global high table both on the origin of the virus as well as the role of the WHO in handling of the virus. Until now, India had maintained a neutral stand on the issue. While on the Taiwan issue, India has yet not made its decision public. However, India is playing its cards with caution given that the choice is strongly informed by Sino-US dynamics. What puts India in a fix is the quandary of US pressure to act responsibly concomitant with Chinese pressure to comply to the diplomatic commitment towards the "One-China Principle".[35] Hence, in the post-COVID world, India will have to make some tough choices to secure its seat at the high table.

II. India in the Global Value Chain System

COVID-19 has severely disrupted the export-import supply chain, resulting from decline in Chinese exports and imports into China from other countries due to the pandemic. The fallout effect of which has surfaced the global need to diversify the supply chain by reducing the dependency on China and China-based manufacturing- the 'World's Factory'. With countries choosing to 'exit China', India is in a position to benefit from a potential shift in the global supply chain away from China—becoming the world's 'new preferred' destination for investment. What makes India a preferred choice is the large size of its market and most importantly, cheap cost of labour. To note, Apple is gradually shifting its manufacturing units to other countries, beginning with setting up a manufacturing base in collaboration with Foxconn in

India. While South Korea's Samsung has closed operations in China and relocated manufacturing units to India, other than Vietnam.

It is also reported that about 1,000 foreign companies are in discussion with the Indian authorities, of which, 300 are in active pursuit of production plans in sectors such as mobiles, electronics, medical devices, textiles and synthetic fibre.[36] Enterprises from countries including Japan, USA and South Korea, have expressed interest in relocating to India.[37] Catering to the growing global demand of investment in India, New Delhi too is undertaking required policy measures to facilitate this possibility amidst the pandemic. To seize the opportunity, India is reported to have identified land parcels across the country spanning 461,589 hectares—almost the size of Luxembourg—in support of these anticipated investments.[38] India's action comes as a welcoming measure for foreign companies against the longstanding issue of 'land acquisition'—one of the biggest impediments for companies looking to invest in India. This highlights the fact that India is gradually changing its old mindset and opting for relaxation of conditions to ease the process of 'doing business in India', which has been China's strongest credential.

However, the challenge for India lies in pitching a strong case given it has other potential competitors such as Vietnam, Thailand, Bangladesh, Taiwan, Cambodia and the Philippines which too offer cheap labour. Among them, Vietnam appears to be India's biggest competition as Hanoi is being seen as a "safe investment destination" after COVID-19.[39] Vietnam is attracting foreign investment with high-tech and high benefit projects mainly expected in four industries: information technology and high technology, electronic equipment, e-commerce and logistics, and consumer goods and retail.[40]

With the pandemic providing a one-time opportunity, India needs to capitalise on the demand from international manufacturers that are intending to diversify their supply chains away from China. With other Asian countries already in competition, India needs to pitch its case strong both in terms of credibility as well as sustainability. Hence, India cannot afford to miss the bus.

III. India Steering the Regional Wheel of Influence—SAARC and Indo-Pacific

The other frontier that provides India with an opportunity to magnify its global role is the SAARC and Indo-Pacific. As already noted in Modi's virtual diplomacy with SAARC in response to the pandemic, the impetus has been set to steer the wheel forward—getting SAARC back on a running track. India has already highlighted its responsive attitude towards its immediate neighbourhood through medical diplomacy. In addition, India has also displayed its responsible behaviour towards its extended neighbourhood—in the Indo-Pacific Region. New Delhi's diplomatic outreach predominantly catered to the Indian Ocean countries, as seen in sending aid from SAARC countries to that of reaching Mauritius and Seychelles in the Western Indian Ocean. There is little doubt on the emerging role of India not just as a key player but also as a responsible actor in the Indo-Pacific.

Amidst the pandemic, India has already set its footprints in the region that calls for a bigger and influential role in the post-COVID world. This will provide a boost to India's strategic interests in the region, such as: first, provide New Delhi with an opportunity to rise above its long labelled 'middle-power' status, added with close strategic relationship with the USA and its allies in the region. This will significantly add to India's great power aspirations and power projections both in the Indo-Pacific region as well on the globe at large. Second, provide an upthrust to India's Act East Policy as well as the Extended Neighbourhood Policy. Third, act as a counter-balance to China's growing footprints in the Indian Ocean. Fourth, provide a stronger push to the India-US Strategic Partnership, mainly in defence ties. Adding to the agreements such as 2016 Logistics Exchange Memorandum of Agreement (LEMOA) and 2018 Communications Compatibility and Security Agreement (COMCASA), the defence ties will get a further impetus from arms transfer, increased military exercise, such as Tiger Triumph, the first bilateral tri-service amphibious military exercise between the USA and India since 2019; and the possibility of being party to the Blue Dot Network, an alternative to counter China's Belt and Road Initiative. Lastly, it will further boost India-Australia relations, which has been recently upgraded to a Comprehensive

Strategic Partnership signed under nine arrangements that includes 'mutual logistics support' for their militaries.

Hence, the post-pandemic world would not let India to remain low key. It will rather push India to tap on its potential to take charge in the regional spheres of influence.

Conclusion

In an overall assessment, it can be argued that as the pandemic wrecked an unprecedented havoc on the globe, it has also set the stage for a 're-thinking' on matters of international norms and behaviour. The pandemic has raised the debate of the emergence of a 'new world order', defined as the post-COVID world order, wherein, with most countries tilting towards an unfavourable view of China, India on the other hand is witnessing a new dawn in the global arena—not just symbolic—but mainly significant.

Despite its nimble footing, and severity of the COVID-19 situation, India with its goodwill gesture and proactive diplomacy has set its image apart against most of the major powers. Setting a global tone to the handling of the pandemic, India paved its way into the international high club, exemplified by appointment at the WHO; followed by being elected as a non-permanent member of UNSC with vast majority, in the most crucial times. Besides, India's concerted efforts both in its regional neighbourhood and beyond has highlighted its commitment to act as well as lead as a responsive global player. Hence, despite the heavy costs attached to the pandemic, it can also be seen as a 'boon' in disguise, pushing India to claim its long due place in international decision-making. Undoubtedly, in the post-COVID world, India will not just participate but also preside over at the global high table.

NOTES

1 The proposal to appoint India's nominee to the executive board was signed by the 194-nation World Health Assembly. India's Union Health Minister Dr. Harsh Vardhan has succeeded Japan's Dr. Hiroki Nakatani as the Chairman of the Executive Board. In 2019, WHO's South-East Asia group had unanimously decided to elect India's nominee to the executive board for a three-year-term beginning May. The Executive Board decides the agenda for the World Health Assembly meeting.

2 World Health Organization (2020), "WHO Director-General's opening remarks at the media briefing on COVID19. 11 March 2020", 11 March 2020, https://www.who.int/dg/speeches/detail/who-director-general-s-opening-remarks-at-the-media-briefing-on-covid-19—11-march-2020, accessed online 12 May 2020.

3 Quoted in Kallol Bhattacherjee (2020), "Modi calls on SAARC to fight coronavirus", *The Hindu*, 13 March 2020, https://www.thehindu.com/news/national/modi-calls-on-saarc-to-fight-coronavirus/article31059135.ece, accessed online 15 May 2020.

4 Ibid.

5 At the SAARC video conference, the Indian Prime Minister was joined by the Presidents of Afghanistan, Maldives and Sri Lanka; the Prime Ministers of Bangladesh, Nepal and Bhutan, the Minister of State for Health of Pakistan, and the Secretary-General of SAARC.

6 See Ministry of External Affairs, Government of India (2020), "Video Conference of Leaders of SAARC Countries", 16 March 2020, https://mea.gov.in/press-releases.htm?dtl/32540/Video+Conference+of+Leaders+of+SAARC+Countries, accessed online 15 May 2020.

7 Ibid.

8 Capacity building measures through online training modules, establishment of a repository of best practices of dealing with COVID-19 at SAARC Disaster Management Centre, and a website with information in each of the SAARC languages.

9 Ministry of External Affairs, Government of India (2020), "Video Conference", n. 6.

10 See Dipanjan Roy Chaudhury (2020), "India, Saudi Arabia explore virtual G-20 summit to address Covid-19 pandemic", *The Economic Times*, 17 March 2020, https://economictimes.indiatimes.com/news/politics-and-nation/india-saudi-arabia-explore-virtual-g-20-summit-to-address-covid-19-pandemic/articleshow/74679565.cms, accessed online 15 May 2020.

11 The virtual G20 Summit was a culmination of the Finance Ministers and Central Bank Governors Meeting and G20 Sherpas Meeting on the COVID-19 pandemic.

12 G20 Leaders' Statement, Extraordinary G20 Leaders' Summit Statement on COVID-19, https://g20.org/en/media/Documents/G20_Extraordinary%20G20%20Leaders'%20Summit_Statement_EN%20(3).pdf, accessed online 17 May 2020.

13 Ministry of External Affairs, Government of India (2020), "Press Release on the Extraordinary Virtual G20 Leaders' Summit", 26 March 2020, https://www.mea.gov.in/press-releases.htm?dtl/32600/Press_Release_on_the_Extraordinary_Virtual_G20_Leaders_Summit, accessed online 17 May 2020.

14 For details see G20 Saudi Arabia 2020, "Events Calendar", https://g20.org/en/g20/Pages/events.aspx, accessed online 17 May 2020.

15 OECD Interim Economic Assessment, "Coronavirus: The world economy at risk", 2 March 2020, p. 1, https://www.oecd-ilibrary.org/docserver/7969896b-en.pdf?expires=1585314274&id=id&accname=guest&checksum=3973096C22BF163588FC1E0B4E269EE4, accessed online 16 May 2020.

16 See G20 Leaders' Statement, n. 12.

17 The World Bank (2020), "Joint Statement from the World Bank Group and the International Monetary Fund Regarding A Call to Action on the Debt of IDA

Countries", 25 March 2020, https://www.worldbank.org/en/news/statement/2020/03/25/joint-statement-from-the-world-bank-group-and-the-international-monetary-fund-regarding-a-call-to-action-on-the-debt-of-ida-countries, accessed online 17 May 2020.

18 Michael Kugelman (2020), "Narendra Modi's Sisyphean Quest for Global Coronavirus Cooperation", *Foreign Policy*, 30 March 2020, https://foreignpolicy.com/2020/03/30/narendra-modi-india-coronavirus-cooperation/, accessed online 18 May 2020.

19 Shishir Gupta (2020), "India draws up Rs 1 billion Covid-19 medical assistance plan, targets 90 countries", *Hindustan Times*, 11 May 2020, https://www.hindustantimes.com/india-news/india-amps-up-covid-19-medical-assistance-plan-targets-to-reach-90-countries/story-0X1H8z1Zqi9piw6n4 FDu8J.html, accessed online 17 May 2020.

20 Ibid.

21 Ibid.

22 Shishir Gupta (2020), "India dials up medical diplomacy, sends 85 mn HCQ tablets, paracetemol to 108 countries", *Hindustan Times*, 16 April 2020, https://www.hindustantimes.com/india-news/india-dials-up-medical-diplomacy-sending-85-mn-hcq-tablets-to-108-countries/story-O6n44wY3cNKWUcKqKdphGP.html, accessed online 17 May 2020.

23 Ibid.

24 Ibid.

25 Ibid.

26 The 36 nationals belonged to seven countries—Bangladesh (23), Myanmar (2), Maldives (2), China (6), South Africa (1), USA (1) and Madagascar (1).

27 "IAF evacuates 112 from coronavirus-hit Wuhan, Air India repatriates Indian crew from cruise ship", *India Today*, 27 February 2020, https://www.indiatoday.in/india/story/iaf-air-india-flights-evacuate-indians-foreigners-wuhan-japan-ship-1650379-2020-02-27, accessed online 15 May 2020.

28 Huma Siddiqui (2020), "Operation Sanjeevani: India sends 6.7-tonne medical assistance to Maldives amid COVID-19 crisis", *Financial Express*, 02 April 2020, https://www.financialexpress.com/defence/operation-sanjeevani-iaf-airlifts-medical-and-hospital-consumables-for-the-maldives/1917317/, accessed online 17 May 2020.

29 Rezaul H. Laskar (2020), "Govt sends aid to Indian Ocean states", *Hindustan Times*, 11 May 2020, https://www.hindustantimes.com/india-news/govt-sends-aid-to-indian-ocean-states/story-fF7Xfr4tsLoJd1ploCuoyK.html, accessed online 17 May 2020.

30 The proposal is part of a seven-page draft resolution moved by 35 countries and the 27-member European Union. The resolution is being backed by three of the five permanent members of the UN Security Council—UK, Russia and France—along with Japan, Australia, South Korea, New Zealand, South Africa and Turkey, among others. However, both the USA and China are not parties to the resolution. From the SAARC nations, Pakistan, Nepal, Sri Lanka, Maldives and Afghanistan are not signatories to the resolution, except for Bangladesh and Bhutan.

31 Quoted in Shubhajit Roy (2020), "At WHO, India joins 61 nations to seek source of coronavirus", *The Indian Express*, 18 May 2020, https://indianexpress.com/article/

india/at-who-india-joins-61-nations-to-seek-source-of-coronavirus-6414969/, accessed online 19 May 2020.

32 See Ji Rong (2020), *Twitter*, 12 May 2020, https://twitter.com/ChinaSpox_India/status/1260180797165727744, accessed online 18 May 2020.

33 "China opposes arbitrary investigation based on presumption of guilt: Vice FM", *Xinhuanet*, 30 April 2020, http://www.xinhuanet.com/english/2020-04/30/c_139021064.htm, accessed online 18 May 2020.

34 Ministry of Foreign Affairs of the People's Republic of China (2020), "Foreign Ministry Spokesperson Hua Chunying's Regular Press Conference on May 8, 2020", 08 May 2020, https://www.fmprc.gov.cn/mfa_eng/xwfw_665399/s2510_665401/t1777215.shtml, accessed online 18 May 2020.

35 One-China Principle insists that Taiwan is an "inalienable part" of China. It is the foundation stone for the Chinese government's policy on Taiwan. See "Taiwan Question and Reunification of China", http://www.china.org.cn/e-white/taiwan/index.htm, accessed online 17 May 2020.

36 Nirbhay Kumar (2020), "1,000 foreign firms mull production in India, 300 actively pursue plan as 'Exit China' mantra grows", *Business Today*, 22 April 2020, https://www.businesstoday.in/current/economy-politics/1000-foreign-firms-mull-production-in-india-300-actively-pursue-plan-as-exit-china-mantra-grows/story/401462.html, accessed online 19 May 2020.

37 Ibid.

38 Shruti Shrivastava (2020), "India Pledges Easy Access to Land for Factories Leaving China", *Bloomberg*, 04 May 2020, https://www.bloomberg.com/news/articles/2020-05-04/india-offers-land-twice-luxembourg-s-size-to-firms-leaving-china, accessed online 19 May 2020.

39 "Investors consider Viet Nam a safe investment destination after COVID-19", *Viet Nam News*, 23 May 2020, http://bizhub.vn/news/investors-consider-viet-nam-a-safe-investment-destination-after-covid-19_315801.html, accessed online 25 May 2020.

40 Ibid.

5

India's Aye to Eye: State in and State of Surveillance

Akhelesh Bhargava and Kanchana Ramanujam

COVID-19 has created yet another front for India to fight. However, this time the fight is against a deadly virus, with no known cure as of date. Just as WHO classified the virus outbreak as a pandemic, nations worldwide swung into action calling for intense surveillance as a way to prevent and control the spread of COVID-19. The rapid spread of the pandemic has made countries resort to maintaining close surveillance over the people, calling for a global surge of digital surveillance. That is, governments in various countries have employed vast programmes to keep a strict watch on social isolation mechanisms—a measure adopted to 'flatten the curve'. In doing so, countries have enforced mechanisms such as government-sponsored mobile data-tracking apps, apps to record personal contact with others, social-networking sites, closed-circuit television (CCTV) networks equipped with facial recognition, permission schemes to go outside, drones and others. With this phenomenon in place, it can be suggested that until the time a cure or vaccine for COVID-19 is discovered, the surveillance measures will continue to be practised. Given this likelihood, in the post-pandemic situation the growth in surveillance may be hard to scale back.[1]

What is noteworthy is that similar methods have been adopted by countries despite their varied political systems. For instance, the Government of India launched a contact tracing app called "*Aarogya Setu*" keeping users informed if they have been in proximity to COVID-19 patients by scanning a database of known cases of infection.[2] Similarly, in China, citizens are using mandatory health code apps, such as a QR-based health code system by Alipay[3] which is based on a given colour code and determines whether users can travel or leave home.[4] While in Taiwan, phone tracking is being used to help enforce quarantines; Hong Kong issued a StayHomeSafe mobile app, Singapore's TraceTogether app and others[5] to track the spread of the coronavirus. Such mobile phone apps and other electronic surveillance measures may, arguably, violate the fundamental rights and freedoms of citizens, but the situation demands it as surveillance helped to track travellers who hid their travel history and to regulate the restrictions on the movement of people in order to contain the spread of the coronavirus.

What is noteworthy, as compared to others, is that India's *Aarogya Setu* app became the world's fastest app to reach 50 million downloads, an overwhelming response that can be linked to the 'mandatory condition' attached by the Indian government. However, the fallout effect of it was witnessed in the concerns over breach of the right to privacy. On 30 May 2020, India's Ministry of Home Affairs (MHA), while easing lockdown restrictions, removed the 'mandatory' option on the *Aarogya Setu* app, which was earlier a 'must' for every working person in India.[6] In view of this, one can state that COVID-19 has accelerated the process of deploying surveillance mechanisms, providing a boost to India's growing surveillance state.

With these security measures at play, COVID-19 has surfaced as a two-fold perspective of surveillance: at one end, surveillance has emerged as an important mechanism to prevent the spread of the virus. And on the other, it has highlighted the importance of the need to protect data collated in the name of surveillance, thus, making it a 'double-edged sword'.

Given this perspective, the present chapter attempts to elucidate the concept of surveillance, its types and new tools of surveillance in the Information Age. The crux of the chapter lies in examining three key aspects: India's surveillance mechanism, the grey areas in the surveillance architecture, and the ways in which India can correct the existing voids to make its national security more robust.

Surveillance—*Keeping the Watchdog on Alert*

In general, surveillance refers to keeping a round-the-clock watch by human or electronic means on a specific location/area, air-space, water-body, person/people, or an organisation (including its subsidiaries) and people associated with it. It is a systematic ongoing collection, collation, and analysis of data and the timely dissemination of information/synthesised intelligence to those who need to know so that action can be initiated. To aid the process, the Information Age has brought about many new inventions and innovations especially in the field of communication services such as emails, social media networks, and video conferencing. The Internet and satellites have made it possible to see things in real time, serving as tools of surveillance. What is noteworthy is that the aspect of data surveillance[7] has become an integral part of overall surveillance. With the growing security challenges, the advantage lies with the one who is 'the first and the fastest' to access information and able to act on it, as forewarned is forearmed.

With increasing threats to both internal and external security, surveillance has now become a mainstream policy issue while external surveillance involves keeping a close watch on the various war-waging/security-related sources that a neighbouring or distant country could pose. This includes details of the reference country's military capability, terror groups, economic capability, population profile, surveillance and counter-surveillance capabilities, and the like. While internal surveillance refers to keeping the population under watch to the fore, albeit at differing levels, to avoid any form of subversion that poses a threat to national security. This understanding makes it imperative to understand how a state operates surveillance to keep a check on the threats and challenges that can be detrimental to its national security. To note, human surveillance[8] has been one of the primary ways of maintaining checks; however, the advent of technology has expanded the scope, strength and reliability of surveillance. No matter which medium, what lies at the centre is the issue of 'effectiveness'. That is, if one argues for the use of surveillance, then it must be effective in increasing security. Here, effectiveness, as the EU SURVEILLE Project considers, refers to having "the technical capacity to deliver the intended security goals, and when employed for a defined goal within the necessary context achieves the intended outcome".[9]

Surveillance Technology—*The Electronic Eye*

Given the phenomenal improvement and advancement in technology, gadgets such as telephone, radar, camera, and others have made surveillance faster, more penetrating, and accurate. Digital technology has provided the advantage of continuous storage, retrieval and reconstruction of information/intelligence at enhanced speeds, of which, the aerial mode of surveillance has been the most pervasive, accurate and fastest, giving maximum reaction-time to respond to a developing situation. What makes electronic surveillance significant is the use of technology in multitude forms. The various technology enabled devices and mechanisms used for electronic surveillance are:

1. Platforms

These are used for mounting electronic surveillance-devices. They include aircraft, helicopters, ships/boats, hovercrafts, satellites, unmanned aerial vehicles, drones, vehicles, buildings, traffic posts, etc. Drones are evolving continuously and are being miniaturised. These platforms are either custom-built or modified based on the mission.

2. Electronic Gadgets

The gadgets which are mounted/fixed on the above-mentioned platforms have multiple capabilities and may include facilities, such as: being directional/swivel types, having varying sensitivity for sound detection, zooming capability for photo capture, interception capability/ noise generators, lock-on tracking facility for continuous monitoring, stand-alone or networked to central servers, and retrievable or one-time usage, making it an endless list. The modular system of the gadgets makes it possible to increase their capacity depending on the requirement to include reach and duration. These gadgets include radars (to detect aerial/ground objects or human movement), cameras [optical, infra-red (IR), thermal], microphones (dynamic, condenser, ribbon—

with a frequency-range of 80-15000 Hertz), sensors (thermal, acoustics, IR, vibrations), and scanners (full body, vehicle).

3. *Internet and Social Media*

Gaming apps, e-mails, social-media platforms such as Facebook, LinkedIn, WhatsApp and WeChat are widely used and require users to provide their personal data. While these companies may be private, their host countries–the USA and China, have rules in place that makes it compulsory for these companies to share private data with the security agencies on the pretext of 'national security'. Using this data, a profile of an individual can be created over a period of time, without the knowledge of the individual. This is a new form of surveillance.[10]

4. *Mobile Phones and Mobile Apps*

Given the way mobile phones function (working from cell to cell), an individual's movement/location can be easily tracked. Moreover, the network providers are required to maintain records of call data and scripts of conversation.[11] Based on the international mobile equipment identity number,[12] a mobile can be tracked, cloned, blacklisted, and hacked. While mobile tracking apps that have become very popular in recent years can be used to track own security personnel and help in differentiating between friend and foe, however, it has an inherent vulnerability—that of falling into enemy hands. So, while mobile phones have made life very easy, they also pose significant risks to privacy.

With these devices at play, entire communications networks are being placed under surveillance, whether "lawfully," under "voluntary" cooperation arrangements or through state sponsored "hacking".[13] That is to argue, everything is recorded, stored and analysed.

India's Growing Surveillance State

With surveillance technology becoming all pervasive, government surveillance has often faced public scrutiny, with proponents arguing that it increases security, while opponents decry its invasion of privacy.[14] While surveillance technology has proliferated in India as witnessed under the Government's 'Digital India' programme, institutional and legal safeguards have not kept pace. Here, it is important to note that although India has become digital, the social-media control of Indians is in the hands of either the USA or China-based companies, mainly Facebook, Google, Alibaba Group Holdings Limited, Tencent Holdings Limited, etc., and others. Both the Chinese companies (Alibaba and Tencent) have bought millions of dollars worth of stakes in many Indian companies, perhaps motivated by the idea of gaining access to personal data of Indian users. For instance, Alibaba has stakes in Big Basket, Zomato, Snapdeal, Paytm Mall and Paytm; while Tencent Holdings has stakes in Byju's, Dream11, Flipkart, Hike, Ola, Udaan and Swiggy. Here lies the catch-the Indian companies in which they have bought stakes maintain personal data of their subscribers including their *Aadhaar* and credit card numbers.

In this regard, the data collated by these agencies with respect to the Indian population is perhaps much more than what Indian security agencies would have managed to collate over the years. That is to suggest that what rightly should be owned by Indian security agencies are mainly handled by the USA and China. What further adds to the concern is that since digital data can be altered or manipulated, the data received by Indian security forces on request may not be 100 per cent original. This very aspect then gives rise to a serious security concern over exploitation of data.

For instance, given the speculations over China-Pakistan collusion against India, one cannot dismiss the possibility of exploitation of data to create unrest in India. Chinese apps such as Baidu Maps, CamScanner, Oppo Store, PUBG, ShareChat, SHAREit, TikTok, Zoom, and others have become some of the most popular apps in the shortest time, with a huge share provided by 1.3 billion Indians. Through these apps, China has already been able to manipulate Indian citizens into sharing their personal data and also gather information on their likes and dislikes as 'users', very often, pass on security-related data, unwittingly. This then creates serious concerns over one's privacy and data security which then are interlinked to the larger national security dynamics.

Moreover, in the context of COVID-19, a trend to notice is the gradual acquisition of bankrupt global companies by Chinese government-backed companies.[15] To prevent such 'opportunistic takeovers', countries are ring fencing their national interest by setting oversight over foreign investment. Following Australia, Spain and Germany, the Indian government too has passed a law vide Press Note 3 (PN3) that has made foreign investments from countries sharing a 'land border' with India subject to prior government approval.[16] This measure is mainly aimed at restricting Chinese companies' acquisition tendencies. Recently, Facebook (which is of American origin) has bought a 9.99 per cent stake in Jio platforms, a unit of Reliance Industries Ltd (RIL).[17] With this, Facebook will be able to have greater access to the data of Indians.

Therefore, given the security aspects attached, it is important that India focuses on manufacturing its own Smartphones, launches more satellites to make the Indian Regional Navigation Satellite System (IRNSS) more efficient and better than the Global Positioning System (GPS) or Beidou, creates its own user-friendly apps with secured codes, and simultaneously places restrictions on foreign apps with dubious track record. However, at the foremost, India needs to enact a data protection law to protect against the challenges posed by invasive new technologies.

The State of Surveillance in India

I. Keeping an Eye on Targets

Surveillance is imperative for national security and it entails covering various targets. In case of India, to ensure national security through surveillance, the following targets need to be put under a watch:

A. Population

To monitor the population effectively, a National Security Number (NSN), containing all basic data—parents' name, place of birth, current and permanent address, photo (to be updated regularly), facial recognition, 10 finger prints, and iris scan is desired—all saved in a QR code that acts as an operating mechanism. In the case of India, the closest to NSN is the *Aadhaar* number. As on 27 December 2019, it is estimated that 125 crore Indian citizens (over 90 per cent of the population) have an *Aadhaar* number.[18] However, due to privacy concerns, there has been a lot of opposition to the process. The Supreme Court, in a majority opinion, upheld *Aadhaar* as a reasonable restriction on individual privacy that fulfils the government's aim to provide dignity to a large population, declared *Aadhaar* a 'document of empowerment' and 'an unparalleled' identity proof.[19]

B. India's Border

The International Border (IB), the LoC, the Actual Ground Position Line, and the LAC are being manned by security forces to check infiltration. There are gaps in the same that need to be plugged electronically. Weather conditions along India's border are of an extreme nature—cold in the mountains, hot in the desert, and rainy in the North-East. There is no single electronic surveillance device which is suited for all kinds of weather. In view of this, Battlefield Surveillance Radars, acoustic sensors, thermal imagers, mobile communication interceptions including by National Technical Research Organisation (NTRO)-both standalone and networked variety-need to be acquired and deployed. All of them should be connected to local and central processing centres for evaluation and warning. India could learn from Israel's surveillance of the West Bank. This will need a detailed study factoring in the implementation suitable for local conditions.

C. Airspace

The airspace over India, including coastal areas, exclusive economic zones, and island territories is vast. The growth of air traffic including private aircraft has increased substantially in India and is still in the growth phase. In addition, the proliferation of drones pan India, including private owners, has increased exponentially. Though the drone policy has been promulgated, its implementation has not been successful. Therefore, there is a requirement to have a mix of airspace surveillance capability covering different height bands (low, medium, high) and different ranges (short, medium, long). India has already ramped up its drone activity for surveillance in the hinterland, and not just along the borders.[20]

The use of satellites, airborne warning and control systems, surveillance radars, air traffic controllers, reconnaissance aircraft including that of the Aviation Research Centre (ARC), and observation posts are some of the means. All these need to be networked in a common grid using Geographical Reference System. Furthermore, the Indian Air Force's Integrated Air Command and Control System (IACCS) needs to be reworked for the entire country having sectors and sub-sectors.[21] The warning time in case of aerial targets is mostly under a minute. Hence, the sensor to shooter connectivity has to be connected over high bandwidth e-highways. Here, a foolproof, electronic Identification Friend or Foe (IFF) is very essential.

D. Coast Line

India has a 7,520 kilometre-long coastline off the Bay of Bengal in the East, Arabian Sea in the West, and the Indian Ocean in the South, as well as along its many island territories. India also has many river deltas and marshy lands where no one ventures. Infiltration using sea routes has increased worldwide and, therefore, close surveillance of these areas has to be carried out. There are thousands of villages along the coast line and they may become reception areas for infiltrators. The 26/11 Mumbai attacks happened through the sea route. Post that attack, every village has been given a colour-code for all fishing boasts/trawlers for easy detection of infiltrators or alien persons.

In this process, the Indian Navy and the Coast Guard are the principal forces to carry out surveillance of the coast line. During the ongoing COVID-19 pandemic, the Coast Guard has increased surveillance in both the Bay of Bengal and the Arabian Sea.[22] Besides the ships, coastal surveillance radars, electro-optical systems, speed boats, hovercraft, helicopters, and remote operating systems and informers aid in coastal security. All the data links for inputs received are networked for displaying an integrated picture at the regional control centre in real time. That, in turn, is disseminated to allow maximum reaction time for a counter infiltration/smuggling force to act.

II. Grey Areas in India's Security Check

Although India has increasingly upscaled its surveillance system, there still remain some areas that need significant attention to improve the surveillance mechanism. This includes:

First, multiple agencies, each having their own intelligence verticals is an issue. Any input received is seldom shared amongst them due to inter-agency segmentation. There is no common central server where each agency can upload its input or download what has previously been detected/known. All intelligence agencies need to be brought under a uniform accountability code to overcome this lacuna. Second, India, despite having an edge in the fields of satellites and drones, displays a miniscule use of technology as far as surveillance is concerned. In this regard, the revisit time of sub-metre resolution, polar satellites over the target area should be reduced to less than one hour and data links to processing centres and the use of AI is a necessity. Third, India despite being a computer technology powerhouse, yet the security agencies lack technological support. The provision of cloud-based servers, supercomputers with redundancy, AI and data mining, multiple levels of security, etc., are a must in this Information Age. The government needs to invest in this vertical urgently to cope with the ever-increasing load on intelligence agencies. Fourth, lack of funding has greatly affected the timely creation of infrastructure needed for intelligence, such as 'high grade operators' in the field. Fifth, India's large population size makes it challenging to maintain proper checks. More importantly, maintaining the database of the entire population secured then becomes an onerous task. Sixth, given India's porous borders, the illegal, cross-border movement acts a critical issue that needs to be curtailed. There is need to seal these borders physically by fencing and manning, as well as electronically, as insurgent groups usually take advantage of these porous borders.

These existing gaps then call for significant changes in India's surveillance set-up in order to maximise national security.

India's Calling under COVID-19: *Revamp the Surveillance Set-Up*

Surveillance is a serious exercise. In the blink of an eye, an important input can be missed. Two key aspects need to be adhered to: First, with high premium on human capital, the selection of manpower should be done carefully based on the key parameters of dedication and integrity that cannot be compromised in the field of surveillance. For optimum output, the manpower should be put under the scanner regularly. Second, the silo approach to surveillance, which leads to inefficient usage of resources needs to be discarded. Third, all resources should be centrally controlled, both at regional and central levels. Fourth, all vintage equipment should be replaced with the latest gadgets capable of functioning in a stand-alone mode without human interference. Since every equipment requires maintenance, there has to be inbuilt redundancy to ensure continuous coverage. Fifth, whether it is the IB, coastal areas, or airspace, a gap-free grid is desired for effective surveillance.

What is 'Must' in India's To-Do List

Safety of data has become the biggest challenge for the State. The surveillance data stored in servers will be accessed by users. Hackers are active round-the-clock and will go to any length to attack and steal data records. Hence, access by users has to be tightly controlled and secured under multiple levels of security to include physical security with biometrics-based access. The codes for each level should be handled by different teams to prevent subversion. At no time should the codes be compromised as the speed at which the data transfer takes place is in micro and nano seconds. The access to servers for data retrieval should be segmented and only that much data should be allowed access as is necessary. In doing so, India needs to pay attention to the following:

I. Data Handling, Recording and Retrieving

It is clear that 'data' is the future 'oil' for any country. Personal data records and other surveillance-related data have to be digitally stored. The biggest disadvantage of the digital mode of storing is that the data is vulnerable to hacking despite being coded. Hence, India needs to focus on indigenisation and work towards the following:

> (a) Creating multiple servers to store personal data of its citizens with multiple levels/gateways of security; (b) Ensuring in-built tools to detect duplicity by process of iteration; (c) Strengthening the IRNSS by launching additional satellites for redundancy, as well as improving accuracy to sub-metre level. This would ensure that tracking is done based on data from IRNSS rather than GPS; (d) Increasing the number of communication satellites to match the population and requirement of data speed; (e) Promoting manufacture of mobile handsets; (f) Creating in-house data encryption codes to counter hacking; (g) Raising the awareness level of citizens

to restrict them from sharing data on social media platforms of other countries; (h) Creating multiple, social media apps to counter those from the USA and China; (i) Placing restrictions on post-retirement employment of staff working in the security vertical. An undertaking should be obtained from them before they switch jobs, and a code-of-conduct should be spelt out for them; and (j) Undertaking frequent checks on manning personnel for integrity to rule out spying, subversion, or espionage.

II. Creation of Data Command and Control Centres

India needs an integrated command-and-control set-up such as a *Data Command and Control Centre* along with a number of regional data command centres. These centres need to be located in stand-alone buildings having the highest security grade. All centres, both central and regional, have to be star networked on high-speed satellites and optical fibre-based data links with redundancy, and should work in close coordination with each other. Bharat Electronics Limited has created command-and-control centres along the coast for coastal surveillance. These are Coast Guard-specific and they need to be upgraded for multi-service use. Similarly, there is a need to have such centres for intelligence data on population, air traffic, and land border areas. ISRO's fully automated command-and-control centres are worth emulating. The centres should have algorithm-based filters (using specific words or phrases) for data mining and co-opting Big Data Analytics. Each centre should be equipped with supercomputers having computing speed at petafloating point operations per second levels; simply put, quadrillion operations per second.

III. Use of Artificial Intelligence, Algorithms and Deep Data Mining

When the data is in petabytes (2^{50}), it is humanly impossible to search it and get the desired results in a finite time. AI is required to extract information based on statistical parameters, such as specific words or phrases, and carry out correlation. In other words, the processing and evaluation of data is done using computers entirely, with due control being exercised by humans. The speed of the process is dependent on the speed of computers and hence, the requirement for supercomputers. India is lagging far behind in the number of supercomputers and the same needs to be manufactured in-house and exclusively for the purpose of surveillance/intelligence.

IV. Handling Protests against Surveillance

Across the world, many entities and organisations espousing the cause of the 'right to privacy' are countering governments and security agencies. This trend is more pronounced in democratic countries like India. It is appropriate to mention here that individuals share their personal details readily for the purpose of obtaining voter identity cards, bank accounts, passports, driving licences, ration cards, and so forth. They do the same on social media sites, often unwittingly. In fact, while travelling abroad, individuals share personal data, including the purpose of visit and places one intends to visit, with foreign authorities. But, for the purpose of 'national security', there is opposition and protest. However, national interest has to be the core and only guiding factor when it comes to such issues.

Conclusion

Given India's size, its diverse terrain, massive population and despite the resource-crunch, the importance of surveillance can never be overstated. While surveillance of 1.3 billion people may appear daunting, technology has the solution to it. Moreover, the ongoing pandemic has proved how effective surveillance can considerably improve national preparedness against black swan events; thus, significantly aiding national security and making surveillance the need of the hour. Apart from the domestic need, surveillance is also the need of the hour for India to keep a watch on the global exploitation of its data—keeping it restricted and protected. As countries such as the USA and China have ramped up their surveillance and are engaged in massive data collection not only of their citizens, but also on foreign nationals (including Indians) by means of cutting-edge technology, India needs to maintain its own records too.

However, in terms of surveillance, India tends to lag behind significantly—with a huge gap between the desired level and the actual level. This makes it imperative for India to shed its vintage equipment and adopt state-of-the-art technologies capable of functioning in stand-alone mode without human interference. India's intelligence agencies need to ramp up their surveillance procedures, adopt the latest techniques, adapt to information technology and have a centralised control. This calls for an urgent upgrade in India's digital infrastructure, which needs to be oriented towards satellites and optical fibre-based connectivity. In this, indigenisation should become central in improving the surveillance system.

India needs to incorporate the latest technology and broaden its surveillance cover, while simultaneously plugging the holes in existing structures. While privacy concerns remain a pertinent issue, a practical measure can always be drawn to safeguard national interest to secure the nation as a whole. It is time that India invests in such technology-driven surveillance gadgets. The use of technology for recording the minutest detail will eliminate human one-upmanship. The role of organisations such as NTRO, ISRO, etc., is very important in this regard. Thus, the current pandemic has provided India with a window of opportunity to enhance and upgrade its surveillance system, and that should be exploited to the hilt.

NOTES

1 Andrew Roth (2020), "Growth in surveillance may be hard to scale back after Pandemic, experts say", *The Guardian*, 14 April 2020, https://www.theguardian.com/world/2020/apr/14/growth-in-surveillance-may-be-hard-to-scale-back-after-coronavirus-pandemic-experts-say, accessed online 16 May 2020.

2 See Government of India, "Aarogya Setu Mobile App", https://www.mygov.in/aarogya-setu-app/, accessed online 16 May 2020.

3 See Minghe Hu (2020), "Beijing rolls out colour-coded QR system for coronavirus tracking despite concerns over privacy, inaccurate ratings", *South China Morning Post*, 02 March 2020, https://www.scmp.com/tech/apps-social/article/3064574/beijing-rolls-out-colour-coded-qr-system-coronavirus-tracking, accessed online 16 May 2020.

4 Phone apps have been deployed that provide a colour-coded health designation: green, free movement; yellow, seven-day quarantine; red, two-week quarantine and QR code; the codes are based on a person's location, health details and travel history, and therefore, can limit where they can go.

5 For instance, Russia has employed Quick Response (QR) code, CCTV, cameras, mobile phone data, facial recognition, and credit card details as ways to track its populace. In Europe (Brussels, Poland, the Netherlands, Spain, Ireland, and the UK), governments are collecting telecommunication data, employing drones and tracking apps. In the USA, Apple and Google have also acceded to the government's request and tracking apps will run on iPhones and Android phones alike. South

Korea has employed GPS data, CCTV footage, and credit card records to identify and warn suspected victims of the disease.

6 Neetu Chandra Sharma (2020), "Government climbs down on Aarogya Setu by removing mandatory provision", *Livemint*, 30 May 2020, https://www.livemint.com/news/india/government-climbs-down-on-aarogya-setu-by-removing-mandatory-provision-11590850319300.html, accessed online 30 May 2020.

7 Data surveillance is a form of monitoring, conducted to obtain specific data from social media sites or specific applications (apps), without the person knowing about it.

8 This involves gathering intelligence (including trans-border intelligence), prevention and investigation of crimes, protection of a process, person, group or object and the like. It is a slow process requiring trained personnel (spies, data recorders, library custodians, and others) bestowed with the gift of the 'sixth sense' and the ability of piecing bits of data together to produce substantial and actionable information. However, with the evolution of electronic surveillance, the importance of human intelligence cannot be dismissed. For, it is the human brain which can put pieces of input together based on prior knowledge and sequence of action.

9 Quoted in Michelle Cayford and Wolter Pieters (2018), "The effectiveness of surveillance technology: What intelligence officials are saying", *The Information Society*, vol. 34, no. 2, p. 90.

10 Moreover, search-engines are becoming faster by the day, and are capable of locating a name within seconds. If someone has registered anywhere on the Internet, the name will show up.

11 Mobile-network providers are bound by local laws and are required to share any individual's data with security agencies, if need be. The national security agencies, in conjunction with the mobile companies, can listen to every conversation a targeted individual has. This includes details of the person(s) he has contacted or spoken to.

12 It is a unique identification or serial number, normally 15-digits long, that all mobile phones and Smartphones have.

13 Ben Hayes (2014), "State of Surveillance: The NSA Files and the global fightback", in *State of Power 2014*, 06 February 2014, p. 3.

14 Michelle Cayford and Wolter Pieters (2018), "The effectiveness of surveillance technology", n. 9, p. 88.

15 The Chinese policy is very clear—all companies have to share complete data (collated as part of business). This data collected can then be exploited against a country's national interest.

16 Hiren Bhatt and Vikas Pareek (2020), "In times of COVID-19, the rules for national protection against opportunistic investment needs greater clarity", *The Economic Times*, 30 May 2020,https://economictimes.indiatimes.com/small-biz/legal/in-times-of-covid-19-the-rules-for-national-protection-against-opportunist-investment-needs-greater-clarity/articleshow/76104412.cms?from=mdr, accessed online 30 May 2020.

17 "Facebook buys 9.99% stake in Reliance Jio for Rs 43, 574 crore", *The Economic Times*, 23 April 2020, https://economictimes.indiatimes.com/tech/internet/facebook-buys-9-99-stake-in-reliance-jio-for-5-7-billion/articleshow/75283735.cms, accessed online 20 May 2020.

18 "125 Crore Aadhaar Cards Issued Since 2009: Centre", *NDTV.com*, 27 December 2019, https://www.ndtv.com/india-news/centre-says-125-crore-aadhaar-cards-issued-till-date-2155184, accessed online 14 May 2020.

19 Krishnadas Rajagopal (2018), *"Aadhaar gets thumbs up from Supreme Court"*, *The Hindu*, 26 September 2018, https://www.thehindu.com/news/national/aadhaar-gets-thumbs-up-from-supreme-court/article25051538.ece, accessed online 14 May 2020.

20 Every drone needs to be fitted with a radio frequency identification (RFID) chip or a QR code for easy confirmation of owner and rightful use. For drones being used for civilian purposes, it could be made compulsory for the drones to be linked to a mobile tracker app. This will enable security forces to isolate a rogue drone.

21 The system should be pre-fed with own aircraft/aerial objects flight plan data for flight plan correlation. The Directorate General of Civil Aviation should be a subset of IACCS and provide it feeds of all civil aircraft.

22 Naina J.A. (2020), "Coronavirus Lockdown: Indian Coast Guard Ramps Up Surveillance Along Karnataka Coastline, *Deccan Herald*, 19 April 2020, https://www.deccanherald.com/state/top-karnataka-stories/coronavirus-lockdown-indian-coast-guard-ramps-up-surveillance-along-karnataka-coastline-827277.html, accessed online 16 May 2020.

6

India's National Military Strategy: A Task in Hand

Rakesh Sharma

The COVID-19 pandemic with its devastating impact resulting in the economic downfall of countries, the heightened requirements to support the human costs, the overwhelming focus on healthcare spending and the increasing need to get the economy to restart is likely to cause a shift in the priorities of nations. 'Defence expenditure' too is likely to witness a significant impact. Here, the big question is: Will the overwhelming impact of COVID-19 shift the focus away from defence expenditure?

In the pre-COVID phase, as the 2020 SIPRI Report suggests, the global military expenditure exceeded to US$ 1917 billion in 2019, making it the highest since 1988, as shown in Figure 6.1.[1]

Highlighting an increase of 3.6 per cent from 2018 and representing 2.2 per cent of the GDP, the report also exemplifies three key trends:[2] first, it has been the highest level of spending since the 2008 global financial crisis and the largest annual growth in spending since 2010. Second, the 2019 global military expenditure is 7.2 per cent higher than it was in 2010. Third, two Asian countries topped the chart of highest

Figure 6.1: Global Military Expenditure (by Region), 1988-2019

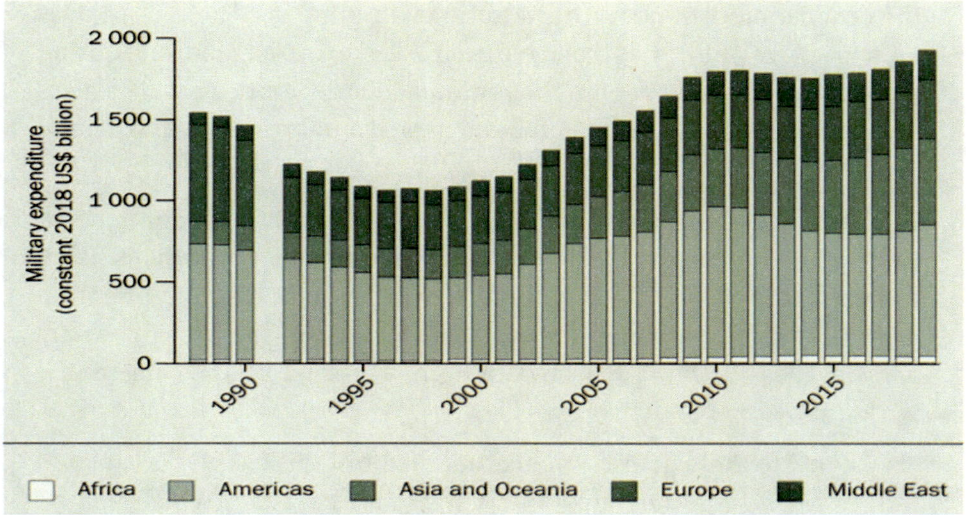

Source: Adapted from SIPRI Military Expenditure Database.[3]

military spending—China and India have ranked second and third respectively after the USA.[4]

Under the debilitating effects of COVID-19, many countries have already announced cuts to their defence budget for the year 2020. However, China, despite being the first and one of the most impacted global economies by the pandemic, has flipped the trend other way. For, at the National People's Congress (NPC), the Chinese leadership increased the military budget to 1.27 trillion Yuan for 2020, a 6.6 per cent rise from 2019 despite the economic decline in the first quarter of the year.[5] This increase further adds to the trend of continuous expansion in the defence expenditure over two decades in the 21st century, as the number has zoomed over 12 times from 107.6 billion Yuan in 1999.[6]

As compared to China, in India, due to the pandemic, the downscaling of the defence budget was imminent. On 1 February 2020, just before the pandemic, India's defence budget for the year 2020-21 was earmarked at Rs. 4,71,378 crore (US$ 66.9 billion), highlighting national security as the top priority of the government.[7] The three Services (Army, Navy and Air Force) have registered a gap of more than Rs. One Lakh Crore between their projected requirements and the

Ministry of Defence's (MoD) allocation, rising committed liabilities and the near certainty of no further additional funding in 2020.[8] The MoD is among several ministries that have been asked to cap expenditure during the first quarter to 20 per cent of its annual budget for this fiscal.[9] This is likely to have a visible effect on India's force modernisation and capital acquisition plans.

With these circumstances at play, it becomes imperative to understand and assess the adversarial environment that India is likely to face in the post-COVID world. The queries that demand attention are: Will this environment remain as status quo of the previous years and decades, or that a newer paradigm is created by the catastrophe wrought by the pandemic?

Owing to these queries, the central theme of this chapter is to assess India's adversarial relations with China and Pakistan, which will be retained in continuity and in foreseeable perpetuity. With continuous military engagement with Pakistan and an impending boundary dispute with China, it is mandatory to explore how New Delhi's relationship with Beijing and Islamabad will unfold. With the warfare in the sub-continent transiting to a modern technological plane, a paradigmatic shift in India's National Military Strategy in the post-pandemic world is highly imminent.

China and Pakistan: India's Never Ending Antagonism

I. The 'Chinese Dream'–Etched in Stone

In November 2012, Chinese President Xi Jinping articulated a vision for the nation's future under the construct of 'Chinese Dream'. The Dream integrates national and personal aspirations, with the twin goals of reclaiming national pride and achieving personal well-being. The fulfilment of the Chinese Dream requires sustained economic growth, expanded equality and an infusion of cultural values to balance materialism. China has nearly reached the pinnacle as a global power with global aspirations, and desires to re-establish its 'Middle-Kingdom' status. To this end, China is spreading its wings; however, contemplating China's future course is "an exercise in frustration".[10]

With a targeted focus to become a 'world class military' by 2050, for

China, the imperative lies in becoming a 'Responsible Great Power'. The 19th Party Congress emphasised that 'China will continue to play the role of a responsible power', which arguably will be unmindful of any likelihood of internal political turmoil, economic decline or international cold war. In this context, would then China's claim to be a 'Responsible Great Power' imply an understanding of the wrath wrought by the pandemic. Does this ensure that the boundary dispute or perceptions of geo-political challenge of a rising India, be a thing of the past. The answer remains 'No'.

The PLA has been active during the pendency of the pandemic on the LAC. Recently, at Naku La in Sikkim, Demchok, Pangong Tso and on the Galwan Nalla in Eastern Ladakh, the PLA had increased transgressions and there have been encounters with Indian Army as witnessed in the violent scuffle at Galwan Valley. Similarly, despite India's protests, on 13 May 2020, the Pakistan government signed a 442-billion Pakistani Rupees (PKR) contract with a joint venture between China Power and the Frontier Works Organization (FWO), a commercial arm of the Pakistani military, for the construction of the Diamer-Bhasha dam in Gilgit-Baltistan (which is Indian territory and presently under Pakistan's occupation).[11] In addition, the 64 billion dollar China-Pakistan Economic Corridor and the expanding Belt and Road Initiative clearly exhibit China's continued ambitious outlook. China, despite the pandemic, remains undeterred.

Chinese actions are deeply rooted in its strategic military guidelines that highlight the need for the PLA to fight and win wars, deter potential adversaries, and secure Chinese national interests overseas. The stress is on the maritime and information domains, offensive air operations, long-distance mobility operations, and space and cyber operations. Informatisation has pre-eminence in PLA's conceptual premise. In a well-planned manner, China is transiting from restructuring, to use of deadly long-range nuclear missiles and questing to become a blue-water navy and acquire potent space and cyber warfare capabilities. With this, China will have a modern military capable of modern war in the future. India can ill-afford to ignore China's increasing economic and military might, its assiduous strategic bases in Indian Ocean Rim nations, lack of progress in the Sino-Indian border talks, and close economic and military affiliations with Pakistan. Thus, India needs to re-vamp itself accordingly.

Hence, COVID-19 has not halted China in the pursuit of its revisionist policies and geo-political ambitions, even by use of force. If the world, wary of China's involvement in the pandemic, were to take strong measures that would significantly put a brake on the 'Chinese Dream'. If so, then China would prepare itself to undertake measures of strong response—also to convey to its own nation. India may then be at the receiving end of PLA's wrath.

China might prefer to portray being a status-quoist responsible power that largely supports largely a benign world order; however, it is increasingly exhibiting signs of revisionism to promote and shape an environment favourable to its ambitions. With increased comprehensive national power and global presence, the possibility of a threat to India manifested by China in the mid and long term cannot be dismissed. Taking a cue from the past, there is a danger that looms large if India fails to comprehend the underpinnings of Chinese behaviour today.

II. Pakistan—Perpetual Crisis in Identity

For Pakistan, a nation without a clear identity, maintaining integrity is an onerous task. It suffers from an identity crisis and has serious internal dissensions. Its internal financial state is precarious, and is under immense pressure from the Financial Action Task Force (FATF) and the Bretton Woods Institutions.

It is primarily the animosity with India (over the Kashmir issue) and Islam that lends Pakistan credence of identity, which is its bedrock to retain itself as a nation-state. It also allows the Pakistan Army with its continual position of eminence in the society. The geo-strategic location of the nation, grave asymmetries in development among the provinces and the extraordinary role that the Army has played is compounded with anxieties on the state of Pakistan—presently and in the future. The fragile state of its economy and the attempts to seek soft loans adds fuel to the fire.

However, Pakistan has always defined its security in tangible terms; need for a military capability to thwart a military threat from India. The twin pillars of the India-centric security perception are building national military capability with the objective of challenging India's military might and providing for an effective defence, and searching for military-oriented alignments, which can assist primarily in dealing with New Delhi.[12] It is also obvious to any discerning analyst that any comprehensive strategic transition to a more benign thinking in Pakistan in the foreseeable future is unlikely, and would keep India embroiled in combating an intransigent Pakistan Army on the LoC and the International Border, along with a proxy war in the hinterland. This kind of hybrid war will give Pakistan distinct advantages. For it, it remains a low cost option, and hampers India's rise as a major power. This makes the Pakistani Army to remain relevant, indispensable and the sole custodian that upholds the Pakistani nation. Pakistan can also test technological weapons like cyber, information, psychological warfare and propaganda, continuously. Pakistan also relies on a modicum of deniability, by describing it as internal dissent in India, and also utilise international fora to publicise human rights violations.

In this context, it is important to recount the Pakistan sponsored-terrorism in Jammu and Kashmir during the pandemic of COVID-19. A major infiltration attempt was made in Keren Sector in J&K in early April 2020, which is not feasible without the direct connivance of Pakistan Army posts. From 15 March to 22 May 2020, there have been 48 incidents of Pakistan-initiated ceasefire violations in J&K along the LoC.[13] In the hinterland, there have been 117 terrorist-initiated incidents from 01 January to 22 May 2020, and 56 militants have been killed in the same period.[14] In addition, the Pakistan Corps Commanders Conference referred to continued support to their designs in J&K, while regular tweets and media briefings at political levels exhibit a status quo attitude. Pakistan's intransigence, hence, to support terrorist organisations and proxy war in J&K even during the ongoing pandemic is well evident.

What adds to India's Pakistan conundrum is the factor of Pakistan-China collusion. That is, Pakistan has already upgraded its security calculus with China through the CPEC—a 15-year plan starting 2015, that is to be completed by 2030. The collusive nuclear warhead-ballistic missile-military hardware nexus between Pakistan and China, described by both as an "all-weather friendship", has grown to menacing proportions. Pakistan has long been a difficult and disruptive neighbour to Afghanistan, hoping to limit India's influence there, and cultivating radical groups within Afghanistan as proxies. It has augmented Afghanistan's instability by providing intelligence, weapons, and protection to the Afghan Taliban and the Haqqani network.[15] Thereby, it can be strongly argued that the anti-India logic will continue to remain the DNA of the Pakistani Army, which virtually controls the polity of the nation, and is unlikely to be done away with within the foreseeable future.

With collusive support from China, Pakistan is also a testing ground for the latest Chinese technology for use in the next conflict or even in peacetime. It would then employ a combination of different types of warfare, conventional, insurgent, terrorist, Information Warfare (IW), a concoction of military and non-military, kinetic and non-kinetic ways of fighting. Hence, any great socio-political change in Pakistan post-pandemic that would lead to an attitudinal change with India may not happen without attendant internal upheaval and instability.

Making of India's National Military Strategy

I. A Politico-Military Responsibility

India has active unsettled borders with both China and Pakistan, and is incessantly countering infiltration and terrorism; hence, bonding between the 'civil' and 'military' is an imperative need. Inevitably, evolution of military strategy is a two-way traffic between the government and military professionals. In a democracy, the final call rests with the government. If Clausewitz's idea that 'war is a continuation of politics by other means' has to be believed, then indeed politicians have the right to dictate on the typology of war. That is to argue, although the armed forces might plan war games and conduct campaigns, the movement and disposition of forces incessantly, in finality have to obtain the political nod.

A military campaign will ever remain to achieve political ends. As a corollary, the Government and the military have to be jointly accountable to the populace for the success or otherwise of the military strategy, in retrospective. It is relevant to mention that under the overarching

National Military Strategy, there may be many military strategies; based on threats and challenges, changing precepts of warfare, ongoing situation; for example in combating insurgencies and terrorism. The National Military Strategy based on envisioned futuristic scenarios, enmeshed with the grand strategy should cumulate utilisation of national power holistically, and may last for a considerable period of time. War fighting strategies would have a reasonable failure rate or achieve less than the envisaged end state. Cases in point are the failure of military strategies of the Maginot Line of the French in World War II, the Bar Lev Line of Israel in the Yom Kippur War and the Blitzkrieg of the Germans against the Soviet Union in 1941. Accordingly, military strategies require in-depth analysis, regularly and especially post war-fighting, to avoid repetition of pitfalls.

Thus, National Military Strategy, not in the operational sense, but in the sense of determining how military means relate to political ends, is a politico-military responsibility. The duty of military leaders is to see that political leaders do not fail because they were inadequately advised or served by soldiers. Politics creates war, so success or failure in war is ultimately the responsibility of the political leadership.[16]

II. Strategic Guidance

National Military Strategy envisages employment of a nation's military capabilities at the highest of levels and requires long-term planning, development and procurement to assure victory or success. If not enunciated in peace; or not planned, developed or trained force created in peace, then inadequacies in the achievement of political aims during a war will rest with the civil-military peacetime imbroglio. More fundamentally, the notion of a separate operational domain simply does not survive contact with reality. As strategic history amply suggests, in cases where soldiers have been given impossible tasks by policy-makers and of soldiers compelled to operate in the absence of clear political guidance.[17]

Hence, to argue further, National Military Strategy derives from a political formulation of national aim, vision and interests, implying the dominant importance of political ends, that is, the National Security Strategy. It is apparent that the NSS would be the bedrock to lead to the development of the National Military Strategy. Again, the military strategy cannot be viewed in isolation, as in prosecution of NSS, the military is one instrument along with other parameters of national power—diplomacy, economic leverages, political strength and national will, cumulated with soft power. Being a singular component of hard power, military power applies force, threatens to do so or becomes an instrument for deterring war.

This conceptualisation denotes creation of a military strategy with sufficient forethought and analysis, and not exactly in the heat of the battle, to achieve the end, with the means at hand, in ways or concepts of employment as pre-decided. Paraphrasing it, military strategy becomes a plan that signifies utilisation of means and concepts of employment of military, to achieve political ends. If prevention of war is the reigning theme of military power, then it has to be proven by enunciation of military doctrines and concepts. Creating requisite military capabilities to operationalise the concepts and to train or exercise in a composite manner to attain military aims which would have been gleaned from political ends. Here, the key is the perceptible political (and national) will and commitment to order execution of military plans. The latter is also part of a psychological mind game. In this formulation, it is apparent that political dynamism is part and parcel of the national security apparatus and peace time planning process for evolving military strategy. Any cleavage in this is bound to be evident by the hesitancy in committal of military power when need be, or in stipulating grave restrictions that would shackle the military in making optimal utilisation of its power.

India's National Military Strategy: *Need for Re-appraisal*

It is well-noted that "[i]n theory, foreign policy determines military strategy. [...] Reality is rarely so simple".[18] To which, National Military Strategy rests on the time-tested equation of 'ends, ways and means'. The national polity, both political and military, will then need to identify the desired ends, by a process that supports effects based on planning for the future. The 'means' are the resources that are required to achieve the ends, such as human resource, force modernisation, technological prowess, weapons systems within the availability of finite budgetary allocations. This process then delineates the imperativeness of minimal to maximum critical capabilities, and establishes the time lines to acquire those.

Nearly US$ 66.9 billion of India's annual defence budget for 2020-21 had been previously allocated, which is nearly 15 per cent of total government expenditure. In the ongoing fiscal year (2020-21), there are already deep budgetary cuts as the call of national socio-economic well-being is rightly taking primacy. This trend is likely to continue for a longer period given the damages incurred by the pandemic. In view of this, it becomes imperative that the oversight to India's defence expenditure is guided by a deeply envisioned and enunciated military strategy—albeit may not be in entirety in the public domain. It becomes axiomatic in this context that specialist structures exist within the larger ambit of political-bureaucratic sphere of influence to partake in creation of India's military strategy.

In this process of preparing the National Military Strategy, it becomes essential for India to take into account its preparation for a modern war against China, and towards Pakistan that is supported by China. In view of this, the strategy in the making should contest the following broad parameters, such as first, Indian nodes and systems may be rendered vulnerable and even incapacitated, which will affect command and control, and cause severe infrastructural damage. This will be by an amalgam of kinetic and non-kinetic warfare, with or without contact of opposing forces. Second, though the PLA may attempt to soften the strong defensive lines across the LAC, in the terrain obtaining, and in the normal prevalent weather conditions, its efficacy is questionable. Hence, warfare may attempt to avoid the defensive strength of the Indian Army, to avoid a slogging match and face large casualties. Territorial aggression across the LAC may only become additional, after significant damage has been wrought by system destruction.

What is important to note is that the formulation of military strategy is a complex bureaucratic-military decision making process translating political goals and contingencies or scenarios into military objectives. In this strategy, the devil lies in the details. In the Clausewitzian 'friction in war', the notion of uncertainty and chance has to be catered for. There is the necessity to possess standing mechanisms that formulate and plan application of the strategy and constantly review, reassess and provide guidelines to further hone the military strategy as is considered obligatory.

What calls for the change? Undoubtedly, prospective wars, whenever prosecuted, will be in multiple domains, some already evident and many off the horizon, in the process of development or under wraps. This makes it important to strategise for disaggregated or aggregated in such a manner that the warfare can be prosecuted. For this, the following broad parameters of strategising become imperative:

First, contested, unsettled borders and territory will remain important contentious issues in future wars, although the larger basis may be related to geo-political rivalries or power struggles. The likelihood of conventional force-on-force kinetic warfare will exist, and must require simultaneous planning. It may be likely that the aggressor (China) utilises a substantially large quantum of force on the territorial frontier of the Tibetan plateau. However, the high altitude and mountainous terrain creates severe restrictions on *ad lib* movement, forced to move through defiles or across plateaus, or utilise the third dimension. Sustenance of force will depend on narrower mountainous axes, aerial drops or makeshift landing grounds. India has the experience and the prowess for defensive and offensive operations in high altitudes. India must plan to offset and defeat the force asymmetry in China's favour by degradation or add a mixture of asymmetric warfare, kinetic strike and defensive layout in tiers. Asymmetric warfare contextually should encompass using linear defended lines only as trip wires, and saturate the battle space with strong deniability by focused and imaginative ruse and subterfuge. Asymmetric warfare in manifold realms would enlarge the battle space to logistical sustenance lines and the forward lines of ingress and choke points as one whole and that will be the key to territorial warfare. Apparently, imaginative asymmetric warfare across the battle space will deny the adversary any technological advantage across the high altitude regions, and stalemate any territorial aggression.

Second, as salience and preparations for modern conventional kinetic war cannot be put on the back burner, substantive offensive capabilities in the form of duly acclimatised, trained and kitted force, must be available for achieving 'across the hump' success and consolidation. Substantial enhancement of third dimension capability will help provide requisite deterrence, and reduce salience on massed combat power.

Third, kinetic and non-kinetic warfare may also go well beyond force-on-force engagement on the territorial sphere as well. It may utilise potent precision guided munitions, hypersonic weaponry, drone swarms, autonomous systems and stealth operational capabilities delivered by multiple modes—ground, air or projectiles. The wars may also be wholly non-kinetic in nature, given the modern warfare domains of information warfare, space, cyber and electronic spectrum that may cripple critical national and defensive infrastructure and forces. This requires India to harden its systems against premature destruction. That is, the Indian Armed Forces need to create a robust, capable, and adaptable operational system of its own to fight a modern war.

The Indian Army needs to focus on acquisition of modern kinetic and non-kinetic capabilities to withstand the onslaught from across the borders, and have offensive capabilities to *quid pro quo* and more. India has to create 'sunrise' offensive kinetic and non-kinetic capabilities across the mountains too, with the corollary that 'sunset' capabilities like linear war fighting will have to be retained at least till mid-term. This modernisation will require India to embrace information warfare technologies, recognising that it will be the application of combinations of technology like processing power, connectivity, machine learning and artificial intelligence, automation, autonomy and quantum computing that will achieve the disruptive effect that India needs. Furthermore, India must develop a framework of strategic capabilities against non-kinetic technological threats, like weaponised information, cyber and other subversive forms of aggression against adversaries. There is a need to accept that multi-domain campaigns will be the future war fighting techniques. Hence, for India, a joint multi-domain specialisation would indicate the right preparation for future warfare.

That brings to the fore, the contemplation of war fighting and hence enunciation of military strategy in an era of a pandemic such as COVID-19. It must be unequivocally stated that with nations reeling from a heavy and serious impact of the pandemic, the initiation of an all-out conventional war is unlikely. Conventional wars, as it is, may be passé! However, operations will have to be undertaken as border skirmishes, as is ongoing at the time of writing in Ladakh, or counter-infiltration/ counter terrorist operations in Kashmir. These operations may get prolonged, and could involve fisticuffs and physical contact. The prophylactic precautions indicated to avoid the spread of the pandemic will be anfractuous in an operational setting, and the likelihood of being consequently infected would exist. This then will be unavoidable fallout of stated military strategy for operations. In time, with the treatment and the vaccine available, suitable compulsory vaccination will obviate the threat of the virus. In the interim, however, during post-military operations, it will be necessary to investigate and test those involved in proximate operations and others in contact, and commence treatment or quarantine protocols. The modus operandi decided to combat the pandemic will also, then, form part of the military strategy for the typology of operations.

Hence, the need of the hour calls for two imperatives: First, given the diverse nature of the Indian Armed Forces, the need lies in requiring a composite, integrated multi-domain task force located regionally/ sectorally, that will amalgamate the sunrise technologies. It cannot be overlooked that sufficient redundancies exist within the armed forces to reconfigure the same, without relying on unnecessary accretions. Second, since logistics is singularly difficult in high-altitude areas, infrastructural resilience with a modern supply chain system are imperative for India. The delivery means must entail aerial support, including drones, to bring about flexibility.

Conclusion

Clausewitz insists that politicians must understand the military instrument that they intend to use. However, in historical practice this has been an exceptional condition, not the norm. In view of this, the coercive actions and policies pursued by China and Pakistan during the course of the pandemic clearly portray the signage of the events to come in the post-pandemic phase. That is to suggest that China would weigh its need as per timing and technological, economic, military and/ or geopolitical coercion. The military coercion against India may lead to a border incident, cause conflicts and infuse instability with the possibility of growing into a major border issue. However, China will choose to be a calculative coercer and may rely on grey zone warfare. In addition, as technology has expanded the domain of warfare to an arena unheard off, such as space, tensions will also arise in new domains. Likewise, information warfare, precision weaponry and autonomous systems and many more will continue to expand to newer vistas. This makes it obvious that the measure of victory in future wars will be the successful paralysis over destruction.

With the security situation in a state of flux under COVID-19, the Indian Armed Forces act as one of the most significant custodians of India's national security. However, in crystallising thoughts and plans on future wars, the time may not be favourable and India might already become the testing ground for military technologies, without even appreciating it. To avoid such a situation, the Indian Armed Forces in concert with the elements of national power need to work to eliminate the strategic and operational uncertainty, and step on the pedal. If the incoming era is of backend warfare, combat by programming computers, launching missiles or operating drone swarms ensconced thousands of miles away, in safe environments, then so be it.

Assuredly, warfare has a future; the all-important question is the typology of warfare, and what it would take to accept it as inevitable, and assiduously work to acquire the capabilities. The strategic conclusion is that technology has fundamentally transformed the character of war, and maybe its nature too, in a significant measure. However, future wars may be without extreme violence, aggression, destruction, and mortality, and yet cause enough suffering to achieve political success.

To sum up, there are momentous changes afoot in the realms of warfare. India's National Military Strategy, in the light of the COVID-19 pandemic, especially in terms of the available means, calls for the need for a structured modernisation. The warfare of the future may well target civilian infrastructure by even non-kinetic means, with the adversary relying on plausible deniability. The nation will demand reprisals, without even clarity on the adversary having employed covert non-kinetic means. Traditional domains of force-on-force would co-exist, but may get reduced in salience. Hence, India's National Military Strategy in the post-COVID era seeks change to create capabilities to fight modern wars, with major influx of technology. The sooner the better, than later!

NOTES

1 Stockholm International Peace Research Institute (2020), "Global military expenditure sees largest annual increase in a decade-says SIPRI-reaching $1917 billion in 2019," 27 April 2020, https://www.sipri.org/research/armament-and-disarmament/arms-and-military-expenditure/military-expenditure, accessed online 15 May 2020.

2 Ibid.

3 Ibid.

4 United States military expenditure reached US$ 732 billion, accounting for 38 per cent of the global military spending. Against this, China's military expenditure reached US$ 261 billion in 2019 and India's spending grew by 6.8 per cent to US$ 71.1 billion accounting for 14 per cent and 3.7 per cent respectively of the global military spending.

5 "Two Sessions 2020: China increases defence spending by 6.6 per cent but sets no GDP target, focuses on Hong Kong national security law", *South China Morning Post*, 22 May 2020, https://www.scmp.com/news/china/politics/article/3085552/two-sessions-2020-live-national-peoples-congress-gets-under-way, accessed online 25 May 2020.

6 Ibid.

7 For details see Laxman Kumar Behera (2020), "India's Defence Budget 2020-2021", IDSA Issue Brief, 04 February 2020, https://idsa.in/system/files/issuebrief/def-bgt-2020-21-040220.pdf, accessed online 18 May 2020.

8 Amit Cowshish (2020), "Defence Sector Reforms: A Long Haul", IDSA Comment, 20 May 2020, https://idsa.in/idsacomments/defence-sector-reforms-amitc-200520, accessed online 22 May 2020.

9 Ibid.

10 Harvey Nelson (2000), "The Future of Chinese State", in David Shambaugh (ed.) *The Modern Chinese State*, Cambridge, UK: Cambridge University Press, p. 216.

11 "Pakistan awards Diamer-Bhasha dam contract of 442 billion PKR to joint venture between Power China and FWO", *The Hindu*, 14 May 2020, https://www.thehindu.com/news/international/pakistan-awards-442bn-diamer-bhasha-dam-contract-to-joint-venture-between-power-china-and-fwo/article31583253.ece, accessed online 20 May 2020.

12 Ayesha Siddiqa (2003), "Pakistan's Security Perspective: Problems of Linearity", in P.R. Kumarswamy (ed.) *Security Beyond Survival*, Sage Publications, New Delhi, p. 169.

13 See South Asian Terrorism Portal, https://www.satp.org/other-data/india-jammukashmir/incidents-of-ceasefire-violations-along-loc-in-JandK_2020, accessed online 18 May 2020.

14 See South Asian Terrorism Portal, https://www.satp.org/datasheet-terrorist-attack/major-incidents/india-jammukashmir, accessed online 18 May 2020.

15 Vanda Felbab-Brown (2018), "Why Pakistan supports terrorist groups, and why the US finds it so hard to induce change", *Brookings*, 05 January 2018, https://www.brookings.edu/blog/order-from-chaos/2018/01/05/why-pakistan-supports-terrorist-groups-and-why-the-us-finds-it-so-hard-to-induce-change, accessed online 20 May 2020.

16 Christopher Bassford (1997), *Policy, Politics, War, and Military Strategy*, http://www.clausewitz.com/readings/Bassford/StrategyDraft/, accessed online 18 May 2020.

17 Colin S. Gray (2007), *War, Peace and International Relations, An Introduction to Strategic History*, Oxon: Routledge, p. 7.

18 Richard K. Betts (1991), *Soldiers, Statesmen and Cold War Crises*, Morning Side Edition, New York, NY: Columbia University Press.

7

Indian Armed Forces: Agile, Responsive and Ever Ready

PK Chakravorty

"The Indian Army, Forever in Battle"

—**Brigadier Gurmeet Kanwal**[1]

The coronavirus in its invisible and constantly mutating mode has transformed the COVID-19 pandemic into a long drawn out war. Just not social-economic stability, but what also needs due attention is the securitisation of nations under the pandemic. For the unpredictability attached to the coronavirus has put all governments across the world into a difficult situation.

The pandemic has affected the Armed Forces of all countries. Currently, the immediate focus is on defensive measures with an aim of keeping personnel fit. However, the Armed Forces have to deal largely with surveillance, diagnosis, offensive and defensive measures. In this regard, the COVID-19 situation has added to the existing internal and external national security threats has placed a high degree of responsibility on the Indian Armed Forces, both in scope and scale.

The Indian Armed Forces are heavily invested in containing the spread of COVID-19 and the pressing concerns for the forces lie in employment of effective strategies to manage the pandemic. In his recent remarks at a IDSA webinar, India's Chief of the Army Staff (COAS) General M. M. Naravane categorically mentioned that the Indian Armed Forces are currently faced with a "two front plus half (terrorism and insurgency) plus half (COVID-19 pandemic) situation".[2] While Admiral Arun Prakash, former Chief of India's Naval Staff, emphasised that the Armed Forces aid to civilian authority must be spontaneous, as was in the tsunami in 2004 when the Indian Navy not only assisted India, but also Sri Lanka, Maldives and Indonesia.[3] Furthermore, he also suggested that the National Disaster Management Authority (NDMA) must jointly plan with the Armed Forces to enable early assessment, guidance and, if need be, assist the country.[4] This brings into perspective the fact that the Indian Armed Forces are simultaneously engaging on two fronts: handling of the pandemic and second, dealing with old security issues vis-à-vis Pakistan and China.

In case of Pakistan, despite its high rate of infection and cases of mortality, it is still heavily investing in infiltrating terrorists into India. In doing so, Pakistan has activated its "deep state" to heat up the environment in Jammu & Kashmir, taking advantage of the Indian Government's focused approach on fighting and controlling COVID-19.[5] This is evident from the heightened cases of ceasefire violations at the LoC as witnessed in infiltration episodes in the Keran sector and Handwara in April 2020. Furthermore, Pakistan is exporting COVID-19 to India by pushing militants infected with virus into Kashmir, as stated by Dilbagh Singh, the Director General of Jammu & Kashmir Police.[6] While on the China front, since early May 2020, India has witnessed two incidents of face-off with the PLA—at 'Finger 4' in Eastern Ladakh and at Nakula in Sikkim. This has been further followed by tensions in the Galwan Nalla and Hot Springs between the Indian Army and the PLA. In response, both the countries have stepped up their military activities by deploying additional troops at the disputed border. In this regard, given the escalating tensions at the India-China border, it is prudent to be vigilant of Chinese activities along the LAC.

With COVID-19 cases on a rise in India despite stringent lockdown measures, it has become far more crucial and essential for the Indian

Armed Forces to be ready to tackle any form of contingency—be it in assisting in containing the pandemic or fighting an adversary. However, with the budgetary cuts due to the coronavirus, the armed forces, as General Naravane stated, will have to maintain its operational efficiency and combat readiness and "remain alive" and cater for the scenario of a "two-front war" with China and Pakistan, even though the possibility is remote.[7]

In this perspective, the aim of this chapter is to understand the role of the Indian Armed Forces under the COVID-19 pandemic. In doing so, it explores two key themes: first, the impact of the pandemic on the Indian Armed Forces; and second, what kind of threats and challenges that Indian Armed Forces should be ready to tackle in the future. Owing to this perspective, the crux of the chapter lies in examining the pandemic from the perspective of 'biological warfare' and its challenges for the Indian Armed Forces.

Indian Armed Forces: *In Action under COVID-19*

In 2018, India's then Defence Minister, Manohar Parrikar, posited that India must be well-prepared to deal with chemical and biological warfare in the wake of changing threat perception and security concerns. He categorically stated that "We [India] should be prepared for any kind of warfare".[8] In a similar vein, under COVID-19, the Indian Armed Forces are engaged in fighting an 'invisible enemy' in the form of a virus. In handling the pandemic, India's Armed Forces have undertaken the following tasks:

First, evacuation of overseas Indians; wherein, on 27 February 2020, 112 Indian citizens and citizens of friendly foreign countries were flown back from Wuhan by the Indian Air Force in a C-17 Globemaster. Further, 58 Indians were evacuated from Tehran on 10 March.[9] While, two of India's naval ships, INS Jalashwa and INS Magar, evacuated Indian citizens from Maldives to India; the first batch of 700 evacuees from Maldives reached India on 10 May.[10]

Second, providing quarantine facilities for the evacuees at seven Army facilitated quarantine centres in Manesar, Jaisalmer, Jodhpur, Chennai, Hindon, Mumbai and Narela in Delhi. In addition, seven other

Air Force quarantine facilities have been kept in a state of readiness in Bhatinda, Devlali, Dundigal, Chakeri, Agra, Gorakhpur and Bengaluru. The Indian Navy has set up quarantine centres at its bases in Vishakapatnam and Kochi. Furthermore, in case of further escalation of the virus crisis, various army schools have also been tasked to be on standby as quarantine facilities.

Third, aiding as medical teams of the Armed Forces Medical Service (AFMS) is acting as the backbone of the Armed Forces' response to the pandemic. More than 8,500 doctors, 50,000 paramedical personnel and the vast infrastructure of the AFMS have been placed at the disposal of the nation. Besides, 51 hospitals with their High Dependency Care Units (HDCU) and Intensive Care Units (ICUs) are being readied to receive patients.

Fourth, boosting self-reliance strategy, as the Armed Forces are re-vamping India's defence production under the "Make in India" initiative instead of importing exorbitant weapon systems. Import of arms is done only to plug critical operational voids until indigenous weapons can be developed.

These proactive measures by the Indian Armed Forces exemplify their steadfast attitude in tackling the pandemic. With fatigue setting in the internal security apparatus such as the Police Force, it becomes imperative for the Indian Armed Forces to be prepared for eventualities.

Evolving Newer Realms of Warfare: *Biological Warfare High on Agenda*

On 27 March 2020, on the occasion of the 45th anniversary of the Biological and Toxin Weapons Convention (BTWC), India underlined the need for international cooperation, including institutional strengthening of the WHO. Given the coronavirus pandemic, India reiterated its call for putting in place a comprehensive and legally binding protocol having a non-discriminatory, verification mechanism to strengthen norms to deal with biological weapons, highlighting the need for an effective response to the challenges posed by new scientific developments in the area.[11] Here, the pertinent query that needs attention is: Is there a possibility of a 'Biological War' being fought under COVID-19?

However, with limited global cooperation, it becomes difficult to reach a definite conclusion based on available facts. However, at a broader level, it can be safely assumed that this can be a combination of Biological Warfare in conjunction with Artificial Intelligence and Information Warfare. This assumption makes it imperative to analyse the component of biological warfare in relation to the COVID-19 pandemic. For numbers as big as 100,000 deaths in the USA compounded with widespread infection globally is tough to ignore, making the situation look like a global war.

Use of biological weapons is not new, and dates back to 400 BC. In World War I, the Germans developed anthrax, glanders, cholera and a wheat fungus and allegedly spread plague in St Petersburg and infected mules with glanders in Mesopotamia. They also attempted to do the same with horses of the French Cavalry. To stop such usage, in 1925, the Geneva Protocol was signed by 108 nations that prohibited the use of chemical and biological weapons in war.[12] Specifically, the Protocol prohibited the use in war of asphyxiating, poisonous or other gases, and of bacteriological methods of warfare.[13] However, this did not stop the use.

During World War II, the Japanese forces operated a secret biological warfare research facility called Unit 731 in Manchuria that carried out human experiments on prisoners. In addition, in post-World War II, biological weapons were used against Vietnam sporadically by the USA from 1960 to 1968. In Vietnam, only one agent was thought likely to be of use, namely, Pneumonic Plague, a highly lethal, highly epidemic disease.[14] It is alleged that the USA decided to conduct a biological war against Vietnam, evident from the report of the WHO.[15]

Furthermore, it was alleged that the erstwhile Soviet Union supplied biological weapons, mainly fungal toxins (Mycotoxins), to government forces to kill dissident tribals and enemy soldiers in Laos, Cambodia and Afghanistan.[16] It is reported that Laos had 6,504 deaths, Cambodia 981 deaths and the casualties caused in Afghanistan are not known.[17] To stop the use of such lethal weapons, in 1972, the Convention on the Prohibition of the Development, Production and Stockpiling of Bacteriological (Biological) and Toxin Weapons and on their Destruction was passed.[18] Currently, 183 countries are signatories to the Convention.

However, the treaty lacks any significant provisions for enforcement or verification. This has enabled a number of signatories to the treaty to maintain active weapons programmes.[19] For instance, Iraq was suspected of having a biological warfare programme in 2003 and Libya was persuaded to terminate its biological programme in 2003. In this context, it becomes essential to comprehend a few issues of the current coronavirus, resulting in a pandemic. To note, the present pandemic was preceded by the SARS epidemic which spread from China in 2002. Then in addition, there was a noted delay from China in informing the WHO. However, unlike COVID-19, SARS, despite the delay, was contained and casualties minimised.[20]

In view of this, Brahma Chellaney has called China "a repeat offender" as it unleashed in a similar manner the world's first 21st-century pandemic, SARS.[21] Chellaney argues that the Communist Party of China (CPC) treated the COVID-19 outbreak in Wuhan in November 2019 as a political embarrassment rather than a public health emergency, delaying the start of containment, tracing, testing and treating until 23 January 2020.[22] In doing so, the CPC has made two mistakes: First, it turned a local outbreak into a global pandemic; and second, China has provided false data of their casualties, which has resulted in a lack of effective response to the pandemic.[23] Furthermore, China also blocked a discussion of the pandemic in the UN Security Council. This aspect of 'lack of transparency' in the handling of the virus outbreak has resulted in the virus taking the form of a pandemic; thus, affecting the entire world, the impact of which is greater than the two World Wars. This makes it imperative to give a serious thought to the issue in order to avoid further casualties.

What makes coronavirus fall under a biological weapons category? Such an intervention is drawn from the finding of French Virologist and Medicine Nobel Laureate Luc Montagnier, who created a scientific firestorm across the world by making a claim that "SARS-CoV-2," is "man-made" as it is the result of an attempt to manufacture a vaccine against the AIDS virus in a Chinese laboratory.[24] In his interview with a French news channel, Montagnier alleged that there was the presence of elements of HIV and malaria in the genome of coronavirus, causing the suspicion that the virus could not have arisen naturally. Although

Montagnier's deductions have been challenged and criticised by a section of the scientific community, his allegations coincides with the timing of the USA calling for a probe into such reports of virus 'leak'. US President Donald Trump in his recent remarks accused China of its "incompetence" and described the pandemic as "mass worldwide killing".[25] Having the highest COVID-19 deaths, the Trump Administration has vehemently called for an independent investigation into the origin of the epidemic in Wuhan in China and Beijing's attempts to conceal the true extent of the epidemic as well as the complicity of the WHO, especially accusing WHO Director General Dr. Tedros Adhanom Ghebreyesus of "missteps" that include abetting China's cover-up.[26]

Although China has consistently resisted an enquiry, on 18 May at the virtual meeting of the World Health Assembly, Chinese President Xi Jinping stated that China supports a "comprehensive evaluation" of the global response to the pandemic, but only after it "has been brought under control".[27] Here, the important aspect to note is that such disasters need to be correctly investigated. For a delayed response on understanding the cause will only delay the cure and thus control of the pandemic.

Biological Weapons: *A Critical Concern for the Future*

Delivery means form an important aspect of biological weapons. There are basically five different types of biological agents: bacteria, rickettsia, viruses, fungi, toxins and Case X genetically engineered virus. These agents can be delivered through two traditional methods. The first is through spray devices and the second is incorporation with the help of explosive devices.[28]

Spray devices entail the use of aerosolised biological agent. Explosive devices include the use of cluster bombs and missile warheads with sub-munitions, while explosive devices were convenient and weak; aerosolised devices were better for dissemination of biological agents. Dissemination rates of efficiency in aerosol systems were in the range of 40-60 per cent whereas in the case of explosive devices the efficiency rate was 1 to 5 per cent.[29] Heat generated by explosive devices during their journey could partially deactivate the biological agent. An aerosol device was a typical bomblet designed for spreading a dried preparation of the agent. The device comprised of a small cylinder of compressed air arranged to direct an air current up through the powdered agent. The clouds that would be generated by aerosol systems would be between 0.5 microns to 10 microns in diameter.[30]

Human beings can also be good delivery agents. Sprayers can be carried on a back pack. Attackers can stand at a distance, attack and then relocate at considerable distance. Attackers are likely to attack, move, reload and attack again and again. This would possibly become a way for terrorist attacks. However, the difficult path is weaponisation. Currently, the technologies for weaponisation have not been integrated. However, over a period of time it would be possible to master these skills.

At the present juncture only a thin wall of terrorist ignorance and inexperience now protects people. However, there is a dangerous category of biological weapons which do not exist in nature waiting in the wings. With the spread of biotechnology and their diversity, it is possible to generate these Case X weapons. It will be more difficult to predict and harder to defend against their use than against pathogens that exist in nature. Preparing for them will be extremely difficult and would involve proactive research.[31]

Indian Armed Forces: *What it has done & What it can do*

I. Prepared to Manage with Budget Cuts

To optimise India's COVID-19 fight and acting on the budgetary cut, the Department of Military Affairs has undertaken the following measures. First, slash expenditure on building of unit medical facilities, training simulators, soldier's cook houses and officers' messes. Second, no concrete garages are to be built hereafter for armoured vehicles like the T-90 Tank. Similarly, Army trucks and jeeps will be housed in temporary sheds. Third, Army, Navy and Air Force to place a hold on purchase of new equipment from the capital budget in the first quarter of this financial year. Fourth, the Army, Navy and Air Force plan to cut down their movements, training exercises as also restructuring their Services to optimise manpower. Force restructuring is being planned to keep the forces primed. The Services will focus on private players and MSMEs to have better equipment with minimum cost. This would help the Armed Forces to continue modernisation despite cuts in allocations. Constant monitoring with innovative ideas would be the answer to this global war.

China has released its defence budget and its modernisation plan continues. The Indian Government is keeping up the modernisation with greater emphasis on Indigenisation. Practically everything will be under Make in India with the private sector having a greater role.

II. Need to Think on the Usage of Biotechnology in Defence

The biotechnological threat is increasing exponentially and there is a need to analyse the threat to get methods to solve the problem. The Indian Armed Forces need to take a fresh look at 'Biotechnology' and its use for military purpose. In the post-COVID period, Indian Armed Forces can undertake the following measures. To suggest, the Department of Military Affairs can form a special project, functioning as a 'Biological Warfare Commission', creating a Biological Warfare Doctrine as also measures to develop Offensive and Defensive Biological Warfare. The Project can be headed by a three-star General and a two-star Medical officer for significant assistance. In addition, the team must comprise a representative each from the three Services, the DRDO, the Ministry of Health, the Ministry of Finance and the Ministry of Defence.

Driven by research, the project must have the capability of knowing the latest viruses and also details of Case X genetically engineered viruses, and to be updated with impending biological weapons and genetically engineered products. Studying the impact on human health conditions is the key and therefore the project must also look at the possibility of agriculture and livestock being harmed and likewise, provide a response mechanism for the same. Furthermore, the Institute of Nuclear Medicine and Allied Sciences (INMAS) and other relevant institutes can also be engaged to aid the process of research. Given the looming uncertainties in the post-pandemic world, India needs to be proactive while dealing with Biological Warfare. India is capable of achieving good results in this field, provided priority and funds are made available. The DRDO must be tasked by the Government to ensure that the project is monitored and a path for success is navigated.

Conclusion

The Indian Armed Forces have always stood by the nation in times of distress and have provided a workable solution on all occasions. COVID-19 is a global pandemic which is similar to a World War. The Armed Forces have played a stellar role in assisting the Government in multifarious tasks during the crisis particularly from the month of March 2020. Currently, the nation is not prepared for Biological Warfare, particularly from attacks by Case X weapons.

The Armed Forces must develop task forces to research on these and also gather intelligence with regard to the spread of such virus, deliberately or accidentally. They should also provide medical assistance and logistical facilities to the nation during multifarious contingencies. Biological Warfare programmes are with 17 nations and it is high time we paid attention to this aspect to develop a proactive approach which will lead us to appropriate defence mechanisms in future. It is recommended that the capabilities of the Armed Forces be used right from the initial stages to minimise pain and casualties

NOTES

1 Gurmeet Kanwal (2008), *Indian Army Vision 2020*, Noida: Harper Collins Publishers, p. 14.

2 Quoted in Rajat Pandit (2020), "Army will maintain combat readiness on fronts with China and Pakistan despite budgetary cuts due to Covid: Gen Naravane", The Times of India, 16 May 2020, https://timesofindia.indiatimes.com/india/army-will-maintain-combat-readiness-on-fronts-with-china-pakistan-despite-budgetary-cuts-due-to-the-coronavirus-pandemic-gen-naravane/articleshow/75762458.cms, accessed online 18 May 2020.

3 "Using the Indian Armed Forces During the COVID-19 Pandemic", Observer Research Foundation, 3 April 2020, https://www.orfonline.org/using-the-indian-armed-forces-during-the-covid-19-pandemic/, accessed online 15 May 2020.

4 Ibid.

5 "How Pakistan deep state is using coronavirus cover to fuel terrorism in Kashmir," *Defence Aviation Post*, 14 May 2020, https://www.defenceaviationpost.com/2020/05/how-pakistan-deep-state-is-using-coronavirus-cover-to-fuel-terrorism-in-kashmir, accessed online 17 May 2020.

6 Quoted in "Pakistan pushing coronavirus infected militants into Kashmir: Jammu & Kashmir DGP", *The Economic Times*, 22 April 2020, https://economictimes.indiatimes.com/news/defence/pakistan-pushing-coronavirus-infected-militants-into-kashmir-jammu-kashmir-dgp/articleshow/75302368.cms, accessed online 18 May 2020.

7 Rajat Pandit (2020), "Army will maintain combat readiness", n. 2.

8 "India must be prepared for biological warfare: Manohar Parrikar", *The Economic Times*, 11 June 2018, https://m.economictimes.com/news/defence/india-must-be-prepared-for-biological-warfare-manohar-parrikar/articleshow/57435338.cms, accessed online 17 May 2020.

9 Dr. (Lt Gen) C. S. Narayanan (2020), "Coronavirus: Armed Forces response to the COVID 19 pandemic in India," *Financial Express*, 22 April 2020, https://www.financialexpress.com/defence/coronavirus-armed-forces-response-to-the-covid-19-pandemic-in-india/1936604/, accessed online 16 May 2020.

10 "First naval ship carrying 700 Indians evacuated from Maldives arrives in Cochin," *The Print*, 10 May 2020, https://theprint.in/india/first-naval-ship-carrying-700-indians-evacuated-from-maldives-arrives-in-cochin/418512/, accessed online 16 May 2020.

11 "Ensure strict compliance of treaty on banning biological weapons: India," *The Economic Times*, 27 March 2020, www.economictimes.indiatimes.com, accessed online 19 May 2020.

12 United Nations, Office for Disarmament Affairs, "1925 Geneva Protocol", https://www.un.org/disarmament/wmd/bio/1925-geneva-protocol/, accessed online 15 May 2020.

13 Ibid.

14 Animesh Roul (2010), "State Actors and Germ Warfare: Historical Perspective, *CBW Magazine*, https://idsa.in/cbwmagazine/StateActorsandGermWarfare_aroul, accessed online 18 May 2020.

15 Ibid.

16 Ibid.

17 Ibid.

18 See, "Convention on the Prohibition of the Development, Production and Stockpiling of Bacteriological (Biological) and Toxin Weapons and on Their Destruction", http://www.opbw.org/convention/conv.html, accessed online 18 May 2020.

19 Mark Schwartz (2001), "Biological warfare an emerging threat to the 21st century", *Stanford News Service*, January 2001, www.news.stanford.edu, accessed online 18 May 2020.

20 Huang Y. (2004), "The SARS Epidemic and its aftermath in China: A Political Perspective," NCBI Bookshelf, www.ncbi.nim.nih.gov, accessed online 18 May 2020.

21 Brahma Chellaney (2020), "China's opacity contributed to spiralling corona infections and deaths. Its geopolitical effects will be long lasting", *The Times of India Blog*, 18 April 2020, https://timesofindia.indiatimes.com/blogs/toi-edit-page/chinas-opacity-contributed-to-spiralling-corona-infections-and-deaths-its-geopolitical-effects-will-be-long-lasting/, accessed online 18 May 2020.

22 Ibid.

23 Ibid.

24 Quoted in Surendra Singh (2020), "Coronavirus man made in Wuhan Lab: Nobel Laureate," *The Times of India*, 19 April 2020, https://timesofindia.indiatimes.com/india/coronavirus-man-made-in-wuhan-lab-nobel-laureate/articleshow/75227989.cms, accessed online 19 May 2020.

25 Yashwant Raj (2020), "Trump calls Covid-19 outbreak 'mass worldwide killing', slams China for 'incompetence," *Hindustan Times*, 20 May 2020, accessed online 20 May 2020.

26 Ibid.

27 Quoted in "China Backs Calls for Probe of COVID Origins - But Not Now", *VOA News*, 18 May 2020, https://www.voanews.com/covid-19-pandemic/china-backs-calls-probe-covid-origins-not-now, accessed online 19 May 2020.

28 Maj Gen (Dr) P. K. Chakraborty (2020), "Biotechnology and Biological Warfare - its Applicability to Indian Armed Forces", Vivekananda International Foundation, 27 April 2020, https://www.vifindia.org/2020/april/27/biotechnology-and-biological-warfare-its-applicability-to-indian-armed-forces%20, accessed online 18 May 2020.

29 Ibid.

30 Ibid.

31 Stefan Riedel (2004), "Biological Warfare and bioterrorism: a Historical Review", Proceedings, October 2004, https://www.ncbi.nlm.nih.gov/pmc/articles/PMC1200679/, accessed online 19 May 2020.

8

India's Quest: To Maximise Security, Exploit Technology

Ashminder Singh Bahal

The consequential effect of the COVID-19 pandemic has brought the entire world to its feet. No major power has been able to predict the magnitude and scope of the virus. With the virus ever evolving, the international community is caught in a quandary over fighting an invisible enemy. Here, the query is: Could technology have helped to warn and predict the spread of the coronavirus? If it could, would the world at large, and India in particular, have suffered any different?

It is important to note that the pandemic has brought the security dynamics to a state of flux. The possibility of a controlled use of a deadly virus with a high degree of inbuilt deniability cannot be dismissed. Rather it might become a norm, which may replace the need for conducting high intensity conflicts (in a nuclear environment), wherein, deniable bio-warfare operations could cause devastating effects on countries without the source ever being proved. For instance, the possibility of bioterrorists carrying deadly virus and spreading it in different areas cannot be ruled out as fiction. In such a scenario, real-time intelligence could play a particularly important role in early detection and prediction wherein, 'technology' acts as the main toolkit, for innovative technologies are making a significant difference in fighting the pandemic.

This brings us to the issue whether the answers lie with technology and can technology be leveraged to become a security maximiser to predict such pandemics in time? Also, can technology act as an enabler to enhance human security in dealing with large-scale effects of bio-warfare? This is to suggest that new security situations under COVID-19 are calling for new changes. It is here that integration of new age technologies such as AI, quantum computing, block chain and internet of things would become imperative. The areas in which advanced technology could be used include detection and early identification of the bio-threat, critical analysis of its impact, predictive determination of its effects detecting lead time available before the threat creates large-scale devastation, surveillance measures to mitigate and monitor its spread, efficient tools and processes to counter or localise it and maintaining the effective functioning of all the elements of society as well as that of the military during the period of threat.

In this perspective, the chapter aims to examine the role of technology in crisis situations. The crux of the paper lies in three key aspects: first, the use of technology to avert a contingency drawn from the larger context of the COVID-19 situation; second, the emerging role of AI in predicting the unpredictable security circumstances and, finally, what India needs to do to upscale its security by usage of technology.

Time's Call: *AI is the New 'Art to Master'*

Artificial Intelligence, dubbed as Industrial Revolution 4.0, is the simulation of human intelligence in machines that are programmed to think like humans, mimic their actions and exhibit traits normally associated with a human being such as learning, reasoning and problem solving.[1] There are two unique characteristics of AI; first, the ability to collect, collate, analyse and interpret data to facilitate taking key decisions such as detection and prediction of a pandemic and second, being autonomous. Autonomous implies the freedom to choose own course of action without human intervention. An AI system such as the neural networks of Google's DeepMind can make connections and reach meanings without relying on pre-defined behavioural algorithms.[2] AI therefore, would be of immense value in handling any form of security situation, be it warfare or a pandemic.

The foremost application of AI lies in Command and Control and decision support. AI technologies provide intelligent computer systems to facilitate decision makers to enhance their speed and effectiveness of decision-making. AI helps in strategic planning and operational tasking. The benefit of using such technologies is that it can provide critical decision support to the appropriate decision-making authority (even pandemic management) when time is short or/and when the number of choices are large. In planning, AI technologies could assist significantly in rapidly analysing the data streamed by the different surveillance and observation platforms and agencies, correlating it with the available characteristics of each input, discerning the correct inputs from the large clutter, predicting the potential spread areas, simulating it on population models and choosing the ideal and appropriate response to prevent the further spread of the pandemic. Furthermore, help to coordinate and supply essential medical services where needed.

Intelligence Agencies & Technology: *Detect, Identify, Risk Assess and Predict*

Intelligence agencies need to play a major role in the detection and identification of pandemics. They need to incorporate Pandemic Detection Cells within their in order to keep a tab on all the bio-labs of hostile nations. This implies that besides the regular sources of intelligence, there is a need to have a central pandemic cell and cells in all the key locations of the hostile countries as well as in the embassies abroad. These cells besides having regular agents and monitoring open information, create AI-based data collection, collation and analytical systems to detect the outbreak of infectious diseases and thereafter undertake risk assessment to monitor and predict its likely spread based on the potential movement of people, goods and services.

It is also important that the system needs to be based on advanced sensors, quantum computing, internet of things and geo-location. Even people would need to be monitored. Controlling a pandemic depends upon our ability to quickly detect, accurately identify, correctly predict the likely areas of spread and then respond effectively to the pandemic.

Intelligence agencies must also collect and analyse telecommunication traffic and social media information obtained through a wide variety of sources. This would not only help in detecting the origin and extent of the pandemic but also help if any rumour or misinformation is being spread.

New technologies provide rapid molecular identification of pathogens and accurate monitoring of disease activity. Web-based surveillance tools and epidemic intelligence techniques facilitate risk assessment and timely outbreak detection.[3] With unprecedented access to data from a wide variety of sources, prediction will come from understanding the movements, behaviour and the touch points of people, once a virus is identified.[4] From the availability of extensive data, we need accurate analysis, so that we can detect its origin, identify its type and analyse its potential spread. This may require quantum computing and use of AI tools. After predicting its source and the potential area of spread, it would be easier to control and manage it.

It was an AI company, Blue Dot, that used machine learning to monitor outbreaks of infectious diseases around the world and was the first to break the news of an outburst of a disease at Wuhan on 30 December 2019.[5] AI is a powerful pattern detection and prediction technology. Machine Learning can currently analyse large volumes of historical data to identify the key variables that can predict and detect a pandemic and its success is dependent on the availability and richness of data fed by data scientists.[6] Hence, the availability of data from a large number of sensors as well as the reliability of the information will be the key to have a rapid intervention system in place to contain pandemics in future. Extensive information is also available in the open domain (Open Source Intelligence); hence, this large amount of data needs to be continuously collected, collated and analysed. This can be efficiently carried out by AI enabled systems.

Surveillance: *New Norm for the Future*

The spread of the pandemic is governed by the movement of people, goods and services. Surveillance is necessary to undertake location tracking as well as monitoring the movement of affected people and warning others who are coming into the vicinity of such persons. Hence, it would require installation of a mobile-based app that is linked to Google Maps to geo-locate every individual with a Smartphone. *Aarogya Setu* is a Smartphone-based mobile application that was developed by the Government of India to connect essential health services with an individual as well as to monitor COVID-19 cases. Here, the caveat lies in the asymmetry between the number of Smartphone users and number of mobiles that have used the application. This makes a large percentage of the Indian population remain undetected. Unless, more people download the app, its effectiveness would be low. Here, it is to be noted that for military personnel, their app network (which should be created) must be on a secure platform and whilst they receive inputs from the government app, they should not provide any information of the movement of military personnel to outside agencies. In this way, they would be alerted if any pandemic-infected person were coming into their vicinity, whilst maintaining operational security. The other limitation is that the quantum of tests in India needs to improve significantly. Currently, India averages just over 100 tests per million.[7]

Besides, there are colour code apps to regulate the movement of citizens, as being used by some countries such as China and Singapore. In addition, integrated CCTV cameras that cover inside and outside areas including roads and streets would prove to be highly valuable in identifying people who come into contact with an infected person. It needs to be ensured that the CCTV cameras installed especially at the streets remain serviceable. This feed needs to be integrated with the pandemic department's central database.

India's New Security Tool Kit: *Things to Have*

I. Drones

In case large areas need to be covered, then perhaps drones are the answer. Pandemic drones could fly overhead, monitor large public spaces, detect people who have fever and even spray areas to kill the pandemic virus. For instance, the University of South Australia has teamed up with Draganfly to develop Pandemic Drones, which use temperature sensors and computer vision to identify symptoms of infectious diseases. The new drones are capable of remotely monitoring temperature, heart and respiratory rate as well as detecting coughing and sneezing at a distance of up to 10m.[8]

Similarly, drones could be used to keep a watch over key areas. Since these are low-flying slow-speed drones, they would be very vulnerable over hostile territory. Surveillance drones were used in China to remind citizens of the quarantine measures and to enforce social-distancing rules.[9] The US Westport Police Department too tested "pandemic drones" to enforce social distancing as well as to monitor the spread of coronavirus.[10]

Drones equipped with loudspeakers are being used to make public announcements to keep people indoors, take necessary precautions, create social-distancing and wear a mask, if stepping outside.[11] When doctors need urgent medical supplies, drones are the fastest means to deliver medical supplies to hospitals and transport samples to laboratories.[12] China adapted drones that were designed to spray pesticides for agricultural applications to spray disinfecting chemicals in public spaces and on epidemic prevention vehicles travelling between impacted areas.[13] This implies that drones in future would not only be used for surveillance and monitoring, but also for transporting medical supplies and samples as well as for spraying disinfectants over large areas. They could also be used to provide essential supplies in key areas. Besides, drones are essential to maintain a close watch along the border and prevent the adversary from gaining tactical advantage while attention is drawn elsewhere, such as India-China tensions along the LAC amidst COVID-19. In addition, drones can be used to keep an eye on terror elements that could be infiltrated in large numbers.

Since complete coverage may be impossible with the help of manned elements, drones could provide a viable solution to it. To this process, AI technologies will not only make drones smart and provide techniques to control them effectively, but also help in identifying hostile elements, prioritising them and then targeting them. A high degree of situational awareness can be achieved by employing a number of smart drones that fly over a wide geographically dispersed contested territory. The significant amount of data that is gathered in the process needs to be processed quickly and analysed accurately. Subsequently, meaningful conclusions can be drawn to facilitate quick decision-making and accelerate the response process; this can only happen, if AI is intimately meshed with drone technology and decision support systems.

Integrating AI technologies completes the detection-identification-response-feedback loop quickly. As technology evolves and computing speed and imaging devices improve, the size of the drones too will continue to reduce resulting in them becoming stealthier, lighter and far more effective. The drones' tasks could be undertaken whilst linked with distant command and control centre that are seamlessly presented with integrated air, land and sea pictures, thereby facilitating efficient and effective decision making and intervention processes. This would need to be supplemented by satellite imagery for monitoring operational changes in deployment and force employment.

II. Robotics in Medical Treatment

Highly contagious viruses require social distancing, even for those who are in the medical profession and who are treating such patients. It is here that robots could play a key role in delivering medical and healthcare and in disinfecting areas. Robots can reduce human contact to a minimum. AI-equipped thermal cameras could also be used to detect temperature variations in a crowd so as to identify those who are infected by the virus. Propeller Technologies, a Tiruchi-based company, unveiled its Zafi Medic robots that are equipped to deliver food and medicines to COVID-19 patients. Asimov Robotics too has developed KARMI-Bot, an autonomous robot that performs functions similar to Zafi, but is also able to disinfect the premises using ultra-violet radiation.[14]

The Danish UVD robot autonomously moves around hospital rooms and operating theatres; covering all critical surfaces with the right amount of UV-C light in order to kill specific viruses. In a typical patient room, 99.99 per cent of all viruses and bacteria are killed within 10 minutes. These robots can also be used at schools, airports and malls.[15] At Wuhan, there are isolation wards that are completely manned by robots that also give medicines to patients. It is therefore important that to clear buildings and office premises, there would be a requirement of procuring robots, especially for critical infrastructure that includes a Command and Control Centre.

III. Social Media, Cyber Operations and AI

During pandemics, misinformation has become a tool to create fear in the minds of the general population so as to demoralise them. This makes it imperative to filter and monitor information available in social media and telecommunication traffic observed in crucial areas. Thereafter, a vast amount of data needs to be analysed quickly and conclusions drawn to identify the spread of misinformation. In doing so, computer vision powered by AI and machine learning as rapidly improving, could help the armed forces and intelligence agencies to accelerate the screening and scouring of vast amounts of data.[16] With social media and other online platforms offering mountains of data on virtually every citizen, AI can be used to detect influencing operations and detect nefarious plots.[17]

In this process, AI-based communication technologies and data analytics could significantly assist in locating, tracking and finally neutralising such elements. It is also seen that when people work from home, chances of cyber attacks increase significantly. The focus here by hostile elements would be to target 'the will' by neutralising our ability to function. It has also been observed that even commercial employees tend to open malicious links and phishing emails. This could end up either corrupting the work environment or leaking secrets. It is here that work from home entails that security protocols be followed. Remote devices such as laptops, wireless and mobile devices, and IoT sensors are highly vulnerable to cyber attacks[18] Machine learning can identify and analyse unknown files and detect cyber threats such as malware so as to prevent the ability of hostile elements to disrupt operations.[19]

AI technologies and systems, while being vulnerable to cyber operations are also enablers that provide protection from cyber warfare. This would therefore, bring in important changes in the way military and civil operations are conducted in the future, which would also imply dominating the cyber dimension at the commencement of any type of warfare including containing pandemics.

IV. Blockchain Technologies

To contain a rapidly spreading pandemic, it is essential that the time from detection to preventing its spread and developing a vaccine be kept to minimum. It is here that blockchain technologies become important. Epidemiologists need high fidelity data to model viruses. The characteristics of blockchain include decentralised management, immutable audit trails, data provenance, data robustness and multiple nodes that are able to share and report vital data instantly.[20] This could be used to improve health care-related processes, such as record management, surveillance, tracking disease outbreaks and managing crisis situations.[21] The use of AI and blockchain technologies results in early detection, effective analysis, quick decision making and provisioning of rapid response. It also helps to identify infected people, isolate clusters, improve diagnostic predictions, detect current location of medical supplies and the nearest treatment centre, provide better treatment and track spreads to newer areas.

Making an Impact: *Training, Simulation and Working in Pandemic Environment*

Perhaps, the most significant impact technologies can make is in simulation, learning, decision making and training. Most predictive models developed for simulating pandemic situations and outcomes rely heavily on AI-based technologies. The effectiveness of such simulation depends on the reliability of data and probabilities that are fed into the simulation models. In simulations, there are many variables that are embedded in the data, which itself is obtained through various sensors and agencies that are tasked to detect the origin of a pandemic and track the movement of people, goods and services. The use of AI and blockchain technology therefore, becomes essential to derive any meaningful learning from such data. Simulations are also required to find vaccines and medicines that cure and prevent the disease from occurring as well as to predict the spread of the disease to newer areas, thereby providing options for taking correct and quick decisions. They could also help in identifying the first responder option once new threats are updated and newer cases are detected or affected people come in contact with the persons who have not yet been exposed to the pandemic.

There would also be a need to carry out simulations to identify measures so that the economic and operational activities can still be conducted, whilst the pandemic containment measures are in force. These would include using virtual systems and technologies dealing with internet of things and quantum computing that help in sharing data and work over secure networks whilst still following pandemic requirements. Training could be carried out using simulation models by providing real-time inputs. An AI-based simulation model typically mimics human intelligence that deals with reasoning, learning, perception creation, planning, language comprehension, problem-solving and decision making.[22] American researchers today are developing AI tools that significantly assist in the conduct of training exercises as well as in deriving meaningful lessons whilst enhancing the safety of trainees.[23] Project Maven of the USA uses computer vision, which is a combination of machine and deep learning, to autonomously find objects of interest,[24] that could give significant training value. These systems help in simulations and in providing effective learning during pandemic times.

Conclusion

Technology can be leveraged to become a security maximiser, both to predict such pandemics in time as well as to act as an enabler to enhance human security. Owing to this perspective, there is a need to create a central pandemic prevention and management department within the PMO coordinated by DMA that will not only identify such threats in time, but also co-ordinate the control of epidemics by utilising appropriate resources from the state agencies.

In drawing lessons from COVID-19, keeping a track of potential pandemic diseases has become imperative for early identification and will help mitigate the destructive effects. To aid this process, robots can be used to reduce the dangers of human contact, AI-equipped thermal cameras can be used to detect temperature variations and identify those who are infected and many other benefits. Furthermore, to minimise the time lost between detection and prevention, blockchain technologies can become significantly useful. These technologies will enhance a state's capability and capacity in terms of early detection, effective analysis, quick decision making and in providing rapid response. Specifically, it will help identify infected people, isolate clusters, improve diagnostic

/www.forbes.com/sites/petertaylor/2020/04/25/could-pandemic-drones-help-slow-coronavirus-probably-not-but-covid-19-is-a-boom-for-business/#46d072a462a4, accessed online 14 May 2020.

11 Mukesh Sharma (2020), "How drones are being used to combat COVID-19", *Geospatial World*, 20 April 2020, https:// www.geospatialworld.net/blogs/how-drones-are-being-used-to-combat-covid-19/, accessed online 14 May 2020.

12 Ibid.

13 Junwei Yang and Timothy Reuter (2020), "3 Ways China is using drones to fight coronavirus", World Economic Forum, 16 March 2020, https://www.weforum.org/agenda/2020/03/three-ways-china-is-using-drones-to-fight-coronavirus/, accessed online 14 May 2020.

14 Nahla Nainar (2020), "Medical Robots to the Rescue in the Battle Against Corona Virus", *The Hindu*, 06 April 2020, https://www.thehindu.com/sci-tech/technology/gadgets/how-medical-robots-are-helping-doctors-in-the-fight-against-coronavirus/article31271989.ece, accessed online 11 May 2020.

15 See, International Federation of Robotics (2020), "IFR Press Releases", 31 March 2020, https://ifr.org/ifr-press-releases/news/robots-help-to-fight-corona-virus-sars-cov-2-worldwide, accessed online 11 May 2020.

16 Alena Kudzko (2018), "Future Now: How AI is Already Changing the Global and Military Landscape", *GLOBSEC*, 06 February 2018, https://www.globsec.org/2018/02/06/future-now-ai-already-changing-global-military-landscape/, accessed online 15 May 2020.

17 Ibid.

18 Heba Soffar (2019), "Military Artificial Intelligence (Military Robots) advantages, disadvantages & applications", *Online Sciences*, 01 June 2019, https://www.online-sciences.com/robotics/military-artificial-intelligence-military-robots-advantages-disadvantages-applications/, accessed online 20 May 2020.

19 Ibid.

20 Carlo R.W.D. Meijer (2020), "Blockchain and Corona Virus: Could It Prevent Future Pandemics', *Finextra*, 24 March 2020, https://www.finextra.com/blogposting/18570/blockchain-and-corona-virus-could-it-prevent-future-pandemics, accessed online 16 May 2020.

21 Ibid.

22 Matt Shipman (2019), "How AI Will Help Train Soldiers in Future", *NC State News*, 02 October 2019, https://news.ncsu.edu/2019/10/ai-training-future-soldiers/, accessed online 17 May 2020.

23 Ibid.

24 See, Sally Cole, "Artificial Intelligence can help warfighters on many fronts", *Military Embedded Systems*, http://mil-embedded.com/articles/artificial-intelligence-help-warfighters-many-fronts/, accessed online 15 May 2020.

9

Making India Future Ready

VK Ahluwalia & Amrita Jash

In pre-COVID phase, the global debates centred on US-China trade war, instability in the Middle East, pressure on Iran, Afghan peace process, complexities in the South China Sea, India-Pakistan tensions and increasing protests worldwide- thus, highlighting the dominant trend of instability caused by state-centric factors. However, the outbreak of COVID-19 replaced these 'high-end concerns' by an all-pervasive 'life-threatening virus' that travelled beyond political boundaries and respected no borders. While the states are prepared for an armed combat, COVID-19 has proved that no sophisticated arms or a high military budget can tackle a life-threatening virus such as SARS-CoV-2. Hence, no country is yet fully prepared.

The reality lies in the fact that the COVID-19 pandemic has declared a global emergency by impacting health, political, economic, social, psychological and security situations, both at the global level as well as within countries. This cataclysmic event has sparked serious concerns resulting in new debates over two pertinent issues: first, what constitutes national security; and second, what should be the preparedness when a state is hit by a life-threatening pandemic, such as the COVID-19. These queries are an outcome of the fact that the invisible virus has dismantled the old perceptions constituting a nation's 'threats and challenges'.

Predominantly focused on handling 'traditional insecurities', the pandemic caught every state off-guard. Despite having the strongest military or the sophisticated technological equipment, the great powers such as the USA, China, UK, EU, and others have failed, not just in preventing the virus from reaching its shores, but more notably, in failing to control the spread of the deadly virus.

This has brought to the fore a few reality checks of the 21st century: first, no country is strong enough to deter a viral attack; second, no economy is strong enough to sustain its growth, and finally, no country can be strong if its people are not safe, in this case, health is the primary concern of security. Therefore, COVID-19 has proved that security interests cannot be coded in the simple binary of 'state and its sovereignty'. The security aspect needs a multi-domain approach, as non-traditional threats today pose a far greater challenge. What lies at the core, is the aspect of human security and well-being of the people. Every nation must realise that its people or human capital is its core strength. Hence, the need of the hour is to 'realign the priorities', such that human security takes precedence in the gamut of national security.

With sanitisation and safety acting as the keywords and social distancing becoming the new norm of behaviour, COVID-19 has led to the emergence of a 'non-contact world'—the 'new normal'. In this new kind of world, states cannot operate in their old ways as the means, ways and even ends of the national security matrix has changed. Therefore, the new dilemma is: What will serve best in the new post-COVID world? The only answer to this is a proactive approach driven by the belief that 'change creates opportunity'. Contextualising it to India, the aim of this chapter is to assess the most pressing concern: 'Is India Future Ready?'

India's COVID-19 experience has brought to the surface the key realities in the handling of the pandemic, mainly: organisational voids, lack of coordinated efforts, an ineffective health care system, lack of understating of the social concerns, the magnitude of migrant labour workforce and its aspirations, and, above all, the preparedness to combat such an all-encompassing emergency inflicted on a dense 1.3 billion population nation. Here, the watchword for India is 'situational preparedness'.

The preceding chapters have already highlighted the issues and concerns that India needs to immediately address. Simplistically put, India is 'not future ready' yet. This reality check makes it imminent to prepare itself for the post-COVID world by drawing lessons from present times and transform challenges into opportunities. For this, India needs to innovate its thought and action. In doing so, providing an overview, the present chapter suggests key recommendations to shape India's preparedness in the post-COVID world.

What India Needs to Do

The recommendations are pivoted on the key objective: How should India respond to the changes? Here, the watchword is 'timely action'. COVID-19's humanitarian crisis is a case of prevailing uncertainty due to delayed and lack of transparent information. The desire is to enhance India's role by prioritising differently, exploiting resources pragmatically and acting proactively to impede any form of national security emergency, including those caused by environmental degradation. For India to be future ready, the need lies in adopting a 'mission-oriented' approach, the guidelines for which are as follows:

I. Organisational Changes: Co-ordination and Integration at all levels

A. At the Apex

- As brought out earlier, a total of 1,307 epidemics were recorded across 172 countries worldwide, between 2011-2017 (WHO report). There is, therefore, a need to either upgrade the National Centre for Disease Control (NCDC) to deal with all facets of such pandemics, or create a separate centralised body directly under the command and control of the PMO. The objective of the Department is to not just identify threats in time and co-ordinate to control them, but to ensure the usage of appropriate resources from different departments/ministries related to health, economy, industry, military, intelligence agencies, national informatics centre and others. The department will act in close coordination with leading organisations such as National Security Council Secretariat (NSCS), the Armed Forces, National Disaster Management Authority (NDMA), Food Safety and

Standards Authority of India (FSSAI), Indian Medical Association (IMA), cyber agencies, industrial chambers (FICCI, CII and others), education and human resources to fight such a contingency.

- A Centre-based 'Migrant Work Force Ministry' should be created, which will function in close coordination with State-based departments in tracking the profile and condition of each migrant labourer. The objective behind this proposed Ministry, in addition to Ministry of Labour and Employment, is to maintain data and meet the aspirations of the over 120 million migrant work force, both within the country and those working abroad. Under the *Atmanirbhar Bharat* mission, the Ministry will undertake skill mapping and help train and build a skilled workforce as required in India's various sectors, making India self-reliant. Here, the *Garib Kalyan Rojgar Yojana* can be instrumental to empower and provide livelihood opportunities to the returnee migrants; while the *Jan Dhan Yojana* can be brought in to effectively deliver micro lending to the workers. Implementation of such schemes on the ground would be the key to success!

B. Enhanced Role of Research and Intelligence Agencies in Detection and Identification

India's Research and Intelligence agencies should establish Pandemic Detection Cells. This will encourage better inter-linkages with the health and appropriate agencies for the provision of early data. Apart from having a central pandemic cell, there should be cells in the key locations of certain select countries (including at embassies abroad). The purpose of these cells will entail obtaining information through appropriate open agencies; monitoring open information; creating AI-based data collection, collation and analyses to detect an outbreak of infectious diseases; and finally, undertake risk assessment to predict the likely spread – at the societal level and through the potential movement of people, goods and services. Intelligence agencies need to ramp-up their surveillance procedures in a coordinated manner, adopt the latest techniques, embrace information technology, and have centralised control. Undoubtedly, an effective intelligence network in biotechnology and biological warfare can save the country from a pandemic and other such calamities.

C. Food Security and Public Distribution System (PDS) Requires Transformation

Food security is one of the most important survival needs of the people. The pandemic and attack by locusts impacted agriculture and production of grains in a few countries. In the future, the world may witness inadequacy of food grains, resulting in sharp increase in food prices. Such conditions will hurt the developing countries the most. Thus, it is critical that global food, health care systems and supply chain of essential items are maintained, albeit with minimum restrictions on tariffs and exports. An accelerated model of air cargoes, shipping, physical inspection, certification, testing, and custom clearances would help to expedite the transaction of goods. What is of significance is the assurance of food supply flows to quarantined areas. It would require cooperation among the countries to facilitate trade and global supply chains to continue by adopting innovative measures. It also requires adequate safeguards by way of biosecurity arrangements, hygiene and sanitation measures during processing of food products, and their distribution chains. To prevent recurrence of criticality in supply of essential items, medical and food items, the countries need to act in greater cooperation while introducing greater transparency and establishing protocols of export restrictions to facilitate trade and flow of goods.

Additionally, the failure of the PDS during COVID-19 led to lakhs of people going hungry, and hence, migrating back to the rural areas. It is to note that India has one of the largest PDS in the world that provides for nearly 800 million people with subsidised grain through a network of fair price shop; however, the allotted grains fail to reach the intended beneficiaries. The entire PDS needs to be examined comprehensively and transformed to cater for such emergencies. A flexible and responsive PDS network, with well laid out emergency action plans, is required to cater for unforeseen surges in demands. Wherein, protecting the marginalised section from rising food prices should be a policy priority. The distribution of food grains and essential items to the rightful beneficiaries to be carried out by conducting unit-level data collection in villages, tehsils, municipalities, and districts rather than focusing at macro-levels or state level.

To aid the process, proper methodologies for micro-level data should be formulated such as the NITI Aayog's December 2019 SDG report. Concentrating on eradication of hunger and poverty at micro-levels is likely to have a multiplier effect on other indicators too in terms of employment generation, and to economically uplift the weaker sections of the society. Here, Aadhaar-linked PDS system should be introduced to collate data of marginalised sections. A similar app such as the *Aarogya Setu* can be created to monitor and track the distribution of Government-sanctioned subsidies and other essential items to the marginalised sections by fair price shops. This will help maintain checks and balances on the overall public distribution system and help curb the problem of middlemen.

D. Data Command and Control Centre

Surveillance is a crucial means to enhance battlefield transparency in an era where the battlefield has expanded into hitherto untouched territories. Given India's population of 1.3 billion, surveillance may look daunting; however, it is important to note that China, despite its massive population has done the same based on national will, improving CCTV coverage, and exploiting technology such as- AI, Facial Recognition, and Big Data Analytics. India has to do something similar in drawing a balance between personal privacy and public safety. Wherein, two important thrust areas for India should entail- enhancing indigenous manufacturing and sensitising the citizenry on cyber hygiene.

In this process, at the bureaucratic level, inter-agency coordination needs to be improved and all sister-agencies should be brought under a common grid. More investment is needed in upgrading the digital infrastructure, increasing the number of communication and remote sensing satellites, and enhancing connectivity through optical fibre networks. To rightly suggest, India needs an integrated command-and-control set-up, such as a Data Command and Control Centre, along with a number of regional data command centres. Furthermore, given India's porous borders and the movement of people, *Aadhaar* number allotted to Indian citizens should be deemed as National Security Number and be made mandatory for all citizens. The number should be linked to a mobile tracking app in order to maintain record of each citizen, while also respecting the freedom of movement and the right to privacy.

Additionally, in future, India may consider use of motorised airborne, waterborne or land-based objects to be e-verifiable by incorporating identification friend-or-foe (IFF) code, radio frequency identification (RFID) chip or quick response (QR) code—to facilitate tracking and monitoring during health emergencies. It is therefore, time that India enhances and upgrades its surveillance system for national security.

II. Prioritising Health in Security Appendix

With direct implications on the survival of human beings, healthcare should be the prime consideration which has traditionally ranked low in the priority list of policy-makers, as reflected in India's minuscule health budget of Rs. 2.6 trillion (1.29 per cent of the GDP) to accommodate 1.3 billion people. Owing to which, COVID-19 cases were an outcome of: high density of population, with greater percentage living in slums and ghettoes; lack of comprehensive data of the population; inadequate medical infrastructure and facilities; untrained staff and insufficient infrastructure; and, ineffective assessment methodology to monitor and record cases. These factors reflect directly on the governing system, leadership, allotment of budget, health care infrastructure and facilities, system of surveillance, monitoring and recording.

To be future ready, India must focus on improving the healthcare facilities with emphasis on greater public-private participation and progressively take the following steps:

- Adopt a **'Universal Health Care Policy'** and which will provide for insurance policies that address epidemics and pandemics.
- Invest in healthcare and infrastructure facilities, indigenous manufacturing of personal protective equipment, protective measures, maintain a database with medical history, create isolation facilities, encourage research on drugs and vaccine development and other health-related R&D to minimise the effects and effectively support a dense population without getting overwhelmed.
- Medical research should be greatly encouraged to boost and bolster the search for a necessary cure for future diseases such as COVID-19. For this, organisations such as the Indian Council of Medical Research need to shift their perspective from mere

production of Western-developed drugs to create and find research-based solutions in India. India must aim to become the **'Pharmacy Hub of the World'**, which will be a booster to India's Medical Tourism Industry, which ranks fifth in the world.

III. Re-booting the Economy by Re-vitalising Indian Industries

It has been proved that only a strong economy can provide security against both traditional and non-traditional security (NTS) threats. However, COVID-19 has called for not just a 'strong economy' but also a 'sustainable strong economy'. This brings into light the fissures in the Indian economy that are weakened by strict regulatory and taxation systems, lack of physical and technological infrastructure, and long drawn bureaucratic procedures. The need lies in increasing the purchasing power of the masses in which credit/loans is one of the measures. However, this will not address the complete problem. The key emphasis should be on development of physical and technological infrastructure and immediate employment measures by rebuilding a sustainable and secure work force. Thereby, to build a sustained economy, India needs to be 'competitive,' with its peers, and thus, adopt the following measures:

- Besides structural reforms and stimulus packages based on priorities, the economy needs to be revived by encouraging and strengthening start-ups, entrepreneurs, banking reforms; increasing demands and purchasing power; abolishing of restrictive laws on labour (as removal only for a few years will not have a lasting impact); export, licensing, and excessive governance that is stifling growth of economic enterprises; and competitive corporate taxes with its peers. However, **'implementation on the ground'** should be central to India's economic strategy.
- The government must work towards overcoming the vulnerabilities in India's 'informal sector' that stood exposed especially after the outbreak of the pandemic. In India, most of the poor people are not digitally connected; therefore, cash-in-hand acts as the utmost priority for survival.
- To support the lower strata, simple reforms such as making

electricity and utility bills free during the pandemic instead of complex concepts such as moratoriums is needed to provide liquidity to the hapless poor. It is an immediate, easy to understand and useful step in re-assuring the common man.

- In the industrial sector, 'Make for India' should become the mantra to help India become self-reliant, self-sufficient, and resilient, and progressively minimise dependency on China and other imports. Success of 'Make in India' would lie in regular monitoring and ensuring performance-based audit. In this process, MSMEs that are the key drivers of the Indian economy, contributing 37.54 per cent of India's GDP, should be revived by the government by innovative means. This sector should be encouraged and supported to make more products indigenously, especially related to electronics, electrical and automobile industries, to curb the dependency on Chinese raw material.
- Sectors such as agriculture, fishing, and poultry, which employ around 70 per cent of the working population, need significant attention. Here, the objective should be to make these sectors self-sustaining largely by providing higher MSPs to support these sectors. Furthermore, the retreating migrant population to the villages should be inducted and employed in these sectors. This will not only ensure security to the affected migrant workforce but also aid the Indian economy and, above all, contribute to food security.
- The usage of digital payment services and home-to-home delivery of essentials through e-commerce platforms has emerged as a useful transaction tool, enhancing India's 'digital' vision. This needs to be further incentivised by developing e-commerce and enabling industries to function online by allowing them to shift sales to online platforms. This will aid the 'contactless situation' under the current pandemic; and most importantly, prevent industries from becoming obsolete or defunct in times of crisis.
- With global companies planning to shift production units out of China, India is provided with an opportunity to accentuate the process in favour of itself. In this regard, immediate reforms

should be carried out to facilitate the ease of doing business in India by reinvigorating the MSME sector. India should be guided by the aim to become a major manufacturing hub, and attract business from the USA, Europe, Japan, and others. In this regard, SEZs need to be further incentivised on priority, by giving tax exemptions/holidays, priority loans, according time-bound approvals with minimal bureaucratic hurdles to encourage industries from investing in these areas. An immediate formulation of policy on this will aid the process of making India a 'preferred investment destination' in attracting companies pulling out from China. This will also significantly step up India's role in the global value and supply chain system.

- India needs to scale up its performance in becoming a leading global player in sectors such as pharmaceuticals, IT, engineering goods, defence equipment, automobiles, agricultural implements, food processing, and other products. This is the need of the hour and India needs to tap on the opportunity.
- India's cottage industries should be provided a significant boost and aided with a stimulus package to produce quality goods, as also to generate employment.

IV. Leading, Engaged and Proactive Foreign Policy & Diplomacy

India needs to act on the opportunity of claiming its rightful role and place as a key stakeholder in the global order. The starting point lies in reviewing diplomatic relations with its immediate and extended neighbourhood. India needs to prioritise its relations with each country and each region, no matter how small or how big. In action, India's foreign policy and diplomacy needs to become far more informed of the global situation, engaged in taking action and ready to take a leading role in global decision-making. For which, India needs to take the following measures:

- Although India's *'Vande Bharat Mission'* to evacuate many stranded Indians from abroad is highly appreciative, the imminent need lies in framing a stringent and rigorous national evacuation policy so that it is not caught off-guard in the future.
- Step up its leadership role in South Asia by providing direction,

support, and expertise in resolving the regional challenges. India needs to take this opportunity in making SAARC functional in both orientation and approach. Given that SAARC is more divided over security interests, health hazards can become a common binding factor to unite the seven nations despite their differences. India with its sophisticated IT, pharmaceutical capability and R&D can take the lead in making South Asia well-equipped to handle such NTS challenges. India can strengthen its strategic influence by taking the lead in finding solutions and building effective capacities to deal with health emergencies that concerns all.

- Step up leadership at the global level by setting new precedents of 'responsible global actor' as the Chairman of the Executive Council of WHO. This is an opportunity that will pave the way for India taking a leading role in global decision-making. Under COVID-19, decisions on human health will indeed take primacy. India should become more active in talks on Climate Change, championing the need for environmental security by making development sustainable and all-encompassing. India needs to make itself heard by taking decisive stands on global issues that are in line with its strategic goals as well as push for its membership at global institutions such as UNSC, Nuclear Suppliers Group (NSG) and others. That notwithstanding, in June 2020, India became a non-permanent member of the UNSC; however, the goal should be to assume permanent membership at UNSC.
- India should become an active player in the global value and supply chain system by building itself as a manufacturing hub supported by a well-networked distribution system. In doing so, India needs to capitalise its cheap labour, resource dividends, market capacity and greater interconnectivity.
- India needs to be timely updated on events and developments taking place not just at its own periphery but also the changing dynamics in West Asia, South China Sea, East China Sea, Hong Kong, Taiwan, and others. It remains indisputable that any form of escalation at any of these quarters will have its implications

on India at all levels—political, economic, diplomatic, and strategic.

- India needs to ramp up its role in the Indian Ocean Region (IOR) and the Indo-Pacific, by progressively improving its capabilities; thus, becoming more visible, active, and responsive as the 'net security provider' and 'the first responder to disasters' in the region. The armed forces and other organisations will accordingly have to be equipped, organised, and trained for such roles.
- India should realign and diversify its relations from trade and investment to that of building greater defence engagements and strategic partnerships with a select number of countries.
- India needs to act vociferously in the creation and joining of G11. This will indeed mark a big step forward in enhancing India's role at the global high table.

V. Tap the Potential of Medical Diplomacy

Although 'Medical Diplomacy' is an emerging field, however, it plays a significant role in serving the dual goals of 'improving global health and bettering international relations' - a way of 'winning heart and minds of people in other countries'. India needs to tap this emerging and potent field of 'Medical Diplomacy' - a humanitarian measure to improve global health but also invariably help to better relations with other countries. It is important to note that India has been engaged in medical diplomacy since the late 1960s; however, India's potential remains untapped. As statistics suggest, India's US$ 30 billion pharmaceutical industry is the largest supplier of generic drugs that accounts for over 20 per cent share of the global supply by volume. In addition, India also fulfils 62 per cent of global demand for vaccines. However, India's heavy dependency on Chinese Active Pharmaceutical Ingredients (APIs), which comprises of 80 per cent by volume, is an area of significant concern. To tackle the issue, in March 2020, Indian government approved a 3 mega bulk Drug Parks; however, it is in the larger interest of India to ensure its timely completion. This will help India to simultaneously emerge as the 'pharmacy hub of the world' as well as a 'net health security provider' —both regionally and globally.

Additionally, a proactive Medical Diplomacy will also serve five core interests: (i) help maintain domestic stability against crisis caused by the spill-over effects of epidemics and natural disasters in regional/ extended neighbourhood (ii) expand the global outreach of Indian pharmaceuticals and provide a significant boost to India's pharmaceutical industry (iii) help globally promote India's traditional medicinal remedies and practices such as *Ayurveda* and *Yoga* (iv) provide an impetus to R&D by encouraging medical start-ups and help export India's medical expertise abroad (v) apart from the civilian engagement, it will help enhance the role and engagement of the Indian Armed Forces Medical Corps in undertaking medical missions beyond the Indian borders. Given these interests, India needs to boost its medical diplomacy in the post-COVID period. This will not only validate India's strong commitment towards 'health security' in its foreign policy with other countries; but also help manage the overlap between military-medical diplomacy.

VI. Defence Preparedness at All Times

In tackling an all-pervasive nature of threats and challenges—external, internal and NTS—it becomes an imperative need for the Indian defence forces **'not to compromise on force preservation and battle readiness'**. As 'force preservation' is the key to battle readiness and operational preparedness, each service should carry out innovative methods to optimise its resources, both in the short-term and long-term perspectives. In this regard, against the pandemic, the following measures need to be considered: 'work from home' to be explored where feasible; 'paperless' culture to be adopted in order to minimise the handling of papers or documents by several personnel; sincere 'attention' to be given to the mental and psychological wellness of soldiers; close combat/training exercises to be minimised; proper quarantine drills to be observed; team sports and group activities to be minimised; and movement of troops outside the cantonments to be restricted – limiting to emergent duties. Concomitantly, this would need a comprehensive review of the existing systems, procedures, training, exercises, human resource management, rationalisation of manpower, ceremonial and administrative needs, capital works, new raisings and equipment, indigenisation, inducting technology enabled systems, and others. The measures to be taken are:

- As Defence Cyber & Space Agencies and Special Operations Division are niche capabilities at strategic-operational levels, these must be developed, as planned.
- Seize the opportunity to carry out structural reforms and transformation of India's Defence Industrial Base (DIB) and Defence Research and Development Organisation (DRDO) by encouraging greater indigenisation and graduating to an 'export-oriented industry' pushed by self-reliance. More specifically, it is time that DRDO, and private home-grown organisations operate with a mission-oriented approach and provide 'cutting edge technologies in select fields' to the Armed Forces to enhance India's reliability and security architecture.
- Although the Defence Testing Infrastructure Scheme (DTIS) launched at an investment of Rs. 400 crores is focussed on boosting the defence sector, however, the biggest challenge to the realisation of the DTIS will be 'system inertia'. This can be tackled by getting the approvals through the bureaucratic chain, release of funds and creation of infrastructure in a mission mode. It is an excellent initiative, which must be monitored to meet the timelines.
- The Armed Forces medical expertise and training can be utilised and put to civil use in times of crisis, such as the pandemic. This will not only fast track treatment of the larger public but also help minimise casualties. In this process, a greater interaction and knowledge-sharing between military and civilian doctors, nurses, and healthcare workers should be encouraged to provide support during emergencies. The armed forces and central armed police forces should identify and earmark biological containment facilities, to facilitate better preparedness during a pandemic or biological attack in any part of the country.
- Although India is a signatory to The Biological Weapons Convention as signed on 15 January 1973, the Indian Armed Forces must pragmatically work out protective and defensive mechanisms to identify and avert any form of a silent biological attack from any adversary or non-state actor in the future. This demands a need to build an effective protective capability to

mitigate biological attacks from foreign and non-state actors. Amidst the pandemic, the possibilities of such future security challenges by implanting 'invisible viruses' cannot be ruled out, wherein, non-state actors are more prone to carry out these tactics of biological warfare than states at large. More specifically, the NDRF and the Armed Forces should develop a capacity to counter all known biological-chemical agents, as in times of crisis they should be the primary responders, along with medical organisations and hospitals. In this, undertaking research on 'weaponisation of virology' would be crucial in making the forces ready to tackle such 'people-centric' contingencies.

- In the long-term perspective, the defence forces must progressively build capabilities of soft, hard, and demonstrated military power to deter threats to its stability and integrity. A strong military muscle deters an adversary to pose threats while combating a pandemic. This is justified by China's transgressions across the LAC in the midst of combating COVID-19 in May-June 2020 and more specifically, the Galwan Valley incident. It is an excellent lesson for the Indian Armed Forces to build a strong military posture, its intelligence and surveillance capabilities, remain vigilant and battle ready against deceitful adversaries even during pandemics. Such tensions not just affect the military but also make the population subjected to a dilemma over perception management, propaganda, and psychological campaign. Indian government and the Armed Forces must make a note of this, and take appropriate measures to counter information campaigns/warfare of the adversary. In doing so, the Armed Forces should build a robust high speed and high bandwidth data communication network capability to always be well-informed, prepared and battle ready.
- India needs to adopt a **'unity of command and unity of purpose'** approach that aids battlefield transparency, situational awareness, and a timely decision and corrective action to any form of ingress. This calls to revisit the *Kargil Review Committee and Group of Ministers Reports (1999-2001)* which recommends structures and systems for robust border management and a responsive intelligence-cum surveillance mechanism to ensure

timely actions. However, the recommendations should be read in keeping with the latest technological changes and systems available in the world.

VII. Finding Solutions to Practical Problems

A. Making Healthcare Affordable and Inclusive

COVID-19's biggest reality check has been lack of health care facilities compounded with a selected approach of treatment; wherein, the plight of common man was felt in inaccessibility to health care as well as increased hospital charges. This very aspect of medical expenditure makes healthcare a privilege. The Government needs to take concrete measures and implement policies to make healthcare accessible and affordable to all. At priority, essential medicines and vaccines should be price controlled with permanent effect. Special medical schemes and health insurance policies should be introduced to handle infectious diseases such as COVID-19. Government hospitals should be upscaled in infrastructure and medical expertise to handle such pandemics. While medical institutes and private hospitals and nursing homes should be prevented from monetising such health emergencies, the government should enact strict laws against making health facilities for-profit business. To cut cost, the existing redundant healthcare units in villages and towns should be revamped and provided with basic medical facilities. Moreover, people in rural areas should be provided with regular awareness on prevention and control of infectious diseases as well as healthy ways of living. In this process, India's pharmaceutical companies can tie up with private hospitals and run routine free health care check-ups in India's hinterlands. This will further aid the process of self-reliant India.

B. Unemployment and Sustainable Induction of Migrant Workforce

The national lockdowns surfaced two key realities: (a) the plight of a non-sustainable migratory workforce; and (b) increasing rate of unemployment, which stands at 24 per cent. As an immediate measure, the government needs to create a separate body to cater to the overwhelming migrant labour population. In addition, some guidelines can be formulated wherein certain minimum labour workforce can always be maintained by major industries to prevent the use of a pandemic as an excuse to lay off workers by employers. Most importantly, to dispel the panic and insecurities as witnessed under the lockdown, the migrant labour workforce should be given certain guarantees in terms of making provisions for minimal wages, accommodation, and medical facilities in times of crisis. Such assurances will not only help retain the workforce, and ensure economic activity, but also help avoid unemployment and migrant exodus.

C. Making Education Sustainable and a Requisite for All

Education in India should not be a privilege of a limited few and needs to have a greater outreach. COVID-19 has made this outreach possible by the use of technology. With virtual classrooms becoming the norm of the future, India needs to take this opportunity to level up its literacy standards by making every village and town digitally connected. In this process, fundamental structural changes in curriculum and syllabi should be made to reinvent the education system-making it eco-friendly, sustainable, R&D and problem-solving oriented.

Progressively, the schools in villages and backward areas can be connected with a city-based school in terms of guidance and knowledge sharing aiding the process of making rural India digitally informed and supported. Vocational training should become part of the regular curriculum to enhance a skilled and self-reliant workforce. Indian youth should be encouraged and supported by the Government in their scientific inventions. Furthermore, the Government should provide low-cost digital devices on a countrywide basis so that no child is left out. In this process, the hinterlands should be given special attention in order to make students from rural areas active contributors to India's future. Wherein, adding to the smart cities, India should take measures to create 'smart villages'—a key requisite in making India future ready to combat any contingency.

With increasing costs attached to privatisation of education, such online and smart ways of learning will not only help reduce the cost but also integrate society at all levels. Furthermore, distance learning can be integrated with online classroom coaching, thus, making the degrees and certificates credible rather than just symbolic.

D. Re-shaping and re-inventing the role of Indian IT Industry

India has an advantage of a strong mix of young Science, Technology, Engineering and Mathematics (SMET) and Management qualified professionals. Capitalising on this professional talent, India can create a competitive edge in development of technology. Indian experts are already heading the world's biggest firms such as Google, Microsoft and others; therefore, the government should encourage young Indian techies and professionals to invent new ways and platforms catering to the new social norms of work from home, virtual classrooms, virtual meetings, cashless transactions and other non-contact ways of working and living. Furthermore, India must build its capacity in creating its own Smartphone technologies, social media networks and indigenous applications as against foreign apps. Thus, providing security against the collection, collation, and handling of data of Indians by foreign bodies.

E. Creating Greater Environmental Awareness and Securing it

Environmental degradation (air pollution, water pollution, etc.) is intricately linked to the health index of a country. As already mentioned in Chapter 1, 1.25 million people die every year in India because of air pollution alone. Therefore, the country needs to allocate an adequate budget and take concrete actions to promote awareness, and prevent adverse effects on the health of its population. The *Swachch Bharat* mission should be strictly adopted at all spectrum of social system. Social awareness in acting responsible towards the environment should be encouraged, practised, and integrated into everyday life. In this process, every school from primary level onwards should have a mandatory course on 'Environmental Problems and Ways to Deal with it'. There should be a special emphasis on India's environmental situation, making students aware and responsible citizens from a very tender age. Afforestation measures should be adopted and 'Green Zones' should be created in residential, workspace and industrial areas. Most importantly, stricter laws on industrial and medical waste management must be formulated to make full use of this natural booster package provided by the ongoing pandemic. The aim should be to create a sustainable way of living by striking a balance with nature.

F. Re-formatting Law and Order

In times of crisis, maintaining law and order becomes a greater necessity. In doing so, there is a need to adopt a humanitarian approach towards problem solving. In drawing lessons from the ongoing pandemic situation, India needs to adopt certain key measures:

- While the Indian Government's current actions to tackle the coronavirus outbreak are guided by the Epidemic Diseases Act, 1897, and the Disaster Management Act, 2005, India needs to draft a modern public health law in the interest of the citizens of India. This should leverage digitisation, self-monitoring, maintaining a nationwide public health and social security database and cater to health education and awareness in times of crisis.
- In the context of COVID-19, fake news, rumour-mongering and misinformation had caused significant fear among the common people, especially the migrant work force and their families, resulting in panic disorder. Accurate information on any form of security and health emergency facing India should be disseminated among the Indian public by the Indian Government or nominated agency(s) in a timely and informed manner. This helps to ward off panic and insecurity amongst common people.
- Irresponsible statements by leaders and media reporting should be put to severe scrutiny and restricted to avoid any form of social dissonance and unrest.
- Every citizen in all strata must be respectful towards the sensitivities of various religions, regions, castes, and ethnic communities to maintain the **'social harmony, integrity, democratic and secular fabric'** of the country.

G. Tap on Frugal Innovation

As the global value and supply chains remain disrupted, access to capital goods and services are the most affected. To provide affordable consumer goods and services to larger section of the population, India should encourage innovation and inexpensive measures to optimally utilise available resources—adding greater value for money and aiding sustainability. However, although *'jugaad'* thinking should be undertaken, but people, talent, technological advancement, innovations, net dividend and leveraging of digitisation should be at the top of the agenda.

H. Creating Social Awareness

One of the ways of taking responsibility is by creating social awareness on issues of concerns. Of which, one of the increasing cause of concern is the mental well-being of the people. As noted, with socio-economic-psychological trauma caused by the pandemic, mental health has emerged as a potent cause of concern. This is highlighted in the increasing rate of suicides, especially among the Indian youth. Therefore, to curb such societal fallouts, it is imminent and should be made mandatory that every institute and sectors of education and work have a counselling facility. More importantly, the societal taboo on 'mental illness and disorders' should be removed by creating greater awareness through promoting mental wellness.

Besides, cleanliness should be advocated by creating awareness on sanitation and hygiene, and thus, facilities for the same should be provided to the common public. Furthermore, awareness on saving water and biodegradable waste management should be strongly promoted. These awareness programmes should be strongly endorsed by the Government at all levels, as it will help build responsible citizens.

Conclusion

In an overall assessment of India's strengths and vulnerabilities, some of these recommendations call for an immediate action-based measures in drafting policy guidelines and standard operating procedures (SOPs) for a 'Future Ready India'. The Government needs to allocate budget and execute the suggestions in a phased manner based on an 'immediate-medium-longterm' goal perspective. Each state should be given a copy of this SOP to be fully prepared in the case of a future pandemic. However, at the heart of the matter lies the practical aspects of living, that the Government needs to deal with in an immediate and effective manner. This entails: lack of medical care; people going hungry due to collapse of PDS; no access to hard money under contactless digital policies (which is only accessible to the privileged, leaving the poor in a vulnerable state); joblessness especially in informal sectors; people stranded due to travel restrictions (road, air, rail, ships); downturn in key industries such as tourism, hospitality, retail, manufacturing, services; and most pressing concerns of the migrant woes caused by unplanned shutdown of various work sectors and the lack of coordination between Centre and the states in making provisions for their safe enroute back home. These issues have highlighted the aspect that old methods of quarantine and isolation cannot cater to a population of 1.3 billion. As is obvious, the safety only accrues to the privileged while more than half of the population is forced to face the challenges of starvation, unemployment, no-cash situation compounded with the burden of lack of heath care facilities and support.

The time to act is now and not give into any further delay. For speedy recovery, the government should work in tandem with private organisations, NGOs, major Think Tanks in the country-maintaining a symbiotic relationship between policymaking and academia. The recovery process demands India to be proactive, agile, informed, responsive and responsible. As only then will India be future ready in terms of safety, security, and sustainability. Therefore, we all are at a moment of nation building and making history.

Notes on Contributors

Lt Gen (Dr.) Rakesh Sharma, PVSM, UYSM, AVSM, VSM (Retd), is Distinguished Fellow at the Centre for Land Warfare Studies. Lt Gen Sharma had commanded a Division in the Jaurian-Akhnoor sector on the LoC, the Fire and Fury Corps in Ladakh, and superannuated as the Adjutant General of the Indian Army. He attended the National Defence College in New Delhi and was a Research Fellow at the Institute of Defence Studies and Analysis. He holds a Ph.D in Defence Studies and is a regular commentator and contributor on national security and defence related issues.

Maj Gen (Dr.) PK Chakravorty, VSM (Retd), is Senior Fellow at the Centre for Land Warfare Studies. He held various prestigious appointments as: former Deputy Director General of Perspective Planning Directorate, Defence Attaché to Vietnam and Additional Director General Artillery at Army Headquarters; and post retirement was an Advisor to BrahMos Aerospace. Maj Gen Chakravorty holds a Ph.D in Defence Technology and is a regular commentator and contributor on issues of geo-strategy, firepower and defence procurement. Maj Gen Chakravorty has authored two books entitled: *Fire Power 2030* (KW Publishers) and *Assessment of Chinese Military Modernisation and its implications for India* (Pentagon Press); and has edited the book on *Future Warfare: Beyond the Horizon* (Pentagon Press).

Air Commodore (Dr.) Ashminder Singh Bahal (Retd), is Distinguished Fellow at the Centre for Land Warfare Studies. Air Commodore Bahal is a gallantry medal recipient Air Force officer and is currently Director at Ministry of Human Resource Development. He was a Distinguished Fellow at USI, Deputy Commandant at College of Air Warfare, Directing Staff at Army War College, Executive Director at Doon Business School, Director at Amity University and diplomat at High Commission of India, Bangladesh. He holds a Ph.D in Political

Science. Air Commodore Bahal has authored the book entitled *Emerging Politico-Security Scenario 2025: Vision for an Emerging Air Force* (Avis Publications).

Brig Akhelesh Bhargava (Retd), is an Army Air Defence (AD) officer. He has commanded a Unit in Western Sector and Eastern Command AD Brigade. He was an Instructor at Army AD College, Director Coordination in Army AD Directorate and Colonel AD (HoA) in Northern Command. Brig Bhargava has keen interest in technology related equipment such as radars, missiles, drones, satellites and electronic warfare. He is a regular contributor to various publications at Centre for Land Warfare Studies.

Col RS Sandhu is Senior Fellow at the Centre for Land Warfare Studies. He is a Gunner Officer from the 9 Para Field Regiment. He is a Paratrooper and an Aviator. Col Sandhu has been awarded the COAS commendation card. He has served in various appointments. Col Sandhu is an alumnus of the prestigious Rashtriya Indian Military Academy. He has a keen interest on issues of national and international politics and security.

Dr. Manjari Singh is Associate Fellow at the Centre for Land Warfare Studies. She holds a Ph.D from Jawaharlal Nehru University. Dr. Singh is a SYLFF Fellow and specialises in sustainable development and the Middle East. She is the Assistant Editor of *Contemporary Review of the Middle East* and Managing Editor of *CLAWS Journal*. Her research papers have appeared in various international journals such as *Migration and Development, Contemporary Review of the Middle East* and *Mediterranean Quarterly* and others. Dr. Singh has co-authored *Persian Gulf 2018: India's Relations with the Region* (Singapore: Palgrave Macmillan); and has co-edited books on: *Islamic Movements in the Middle East: Ideologies, Practices and Political Participation* (New Delhi: Knowledge World) and *National Security Challenges: Young Scholars' Perspective* (CLAWS: Pentagon Press) (forthcoming).

Ms Kanchana Ramanujam has been a Research Assistant at the Centre for Land Warfare Studies. She holds a Bachelor's in Biotechnology (Goa University) and a Master's in Defence and Strategic Studies (University of Madras), and has been a university topper in the latter. Ms Ramanujam was a participant at the *9thXiangshan Forum* in Beijing and has participated in CLAWS' prestigious discussions with Chinese leading Think Tanks such as Academy of Military Sciences and the Shanghai Institutes for International Studies. She has written on issues related to: defence, warfare, China, Pakistan, and technology, especially Biotechnology.

Notes on Editors

Lt Gen (Dr.) VK Ahluwalia, PVSM, AVSM, YSM, VSM (Retd)**, is the Director of Centre for Land Warfare Studies. Lt Gen Ahluwalia superannuated as Army Commander, Central Command in March 2012. As the GOC-in-C, his Division was awarded the *National Green Governance Award (BNHS)* by the Prime Minister of India on 10 November 2005, for conceiving and implementing the unique strategic concept - *'Operation Green Kargil'*. Post retirement as GOC-in-C, he served as a Member in the Armed Forces Tribunal (AFT). The General Officer commanded an infantry brigade, mountain division and corps in Uri- Baramulla, Kargil and Leh-Ladakh sectors respectively. He has also served in the North East and in the states critically affected by the Maoist insurgency in India. Lt Gen Ahluwalia holds a Ph.D in Internal Security and Conflict Resolution. He has authored a book titled *Red Revolution 2020 and beyond* (Bloomsbury India) and has co-edited a book on Kargil titled *Surprise, Strategy and Vijay: 20 years of Kargil and beyond* (Pentagon Press).

Dr. Amrita Jash is Research Fellow and Managing Editor of *CLAWS Journal* at the Centre for Land Warfare Studies. She is a Pavate Fellow and has been a Visiting Fellow at the Department of Politics and International Studies, University of Cambridge. Dr. Jash holds a Ph.D in Chinese Studies from Jawaharlal Nehru University. She has been an Adjunct Faculty at the School of Global Affairs-Ambedkar University Delhi and a Visiting Faculty at the Department of Chinese-Sikkim Central University; a UGC Graduate Fellow (2012-2017); a *US-INDIA-CHINA Initiative* Fellow at *SAIS-Johns Hopkins University* (2013); a researcher under *China's Ministry of Commerce* (2014) and under the *Harvard-Yenching-Nanching Programme* (2015). She has been awarded by the COAS Gen Bipin Rawat for her contribution to Chinese Studies (2019). Dr. Jash's research has appeared in 11 edited books, Peer-Reviewed Journals such as *East Asian Policy, Review of Global Politics, Strategic Analysis, Yonsei Journal, China Report, Maritime Affairs* and *Strategic Vision*. She has published with *CSIS, RUSI, Pacific Forum, RSIS, Think China, Huffington Post, E-IR, Asia Times, Munk School, Crawford School, ISDP, China-India Brief, SADF* and others. Her research expertise are China's foreign policy, strategic and security issues; Chinese military, India-China relations and China-Japan relations.

Index